Praise for Retu.

As a psychiatrist working both with highly successful individuals and with some of the nation's most underserved populations, *Return to Beautiful* makes evident some of the deepest and most important lessons I share with my patients and clients. Look no further; this daring publication by Jelena Petkovic is the perfect demonstration of spiritual, food, lifestyle, and health practices, sure to appeal to those starting their health journeys and those who are deep in their practice. Petkovic expertly leads the way to vibrancy, charisma, and bliss through her transparency, wisdom, insights, and success as a practitioner. Copies of this brave and necessary text will fill my office shelves for sharing at every visit. This book is exactly what my clinic needs.

— **Jonathan Terry**   *DO, ABIHM, Board-certified osteopathic physician and surgeon, general psychiatrist, Diplomate of the American Board of Psychiatry and Neurology (ABPN), Diplomate of the National Board of Physicians and Surgeons (NBPAS), and Diplomate of the American Board of Integrative and Holistic Medicine (ABIHM)*

This book will help you turn back time to a moment in your life you felt your most radiant, joyful, energetic and optimistic! It's your opportunity to feel excited and confident about your health and every aspect of your life. Jelena Petkovic's wisdom, insights, and personal transformation story will shift your perception about aging, life and happiness in general. The content will help remove confusion, frustration and fear around the difficulty of conceiving a life of bliss. This is an opportunity to learn from an innovative medical expert, healer and spiritual leader. Be prepared for more solid, usable, information than you've ever seen inside one book."

— **Nancy Matthews**   *International Speaker, Founder of Women's Prosperity Network*

---

i

Jelena Petkovic has lived, persevered and prospered for years in the world of anti-aging medicine and healing. Her book, *Return to Beautiful*—a distillation of her insights—is written for anyone seeking a strategy to heal not only your body but your life, helping you live in more ease, flow and bliss. This book is sure to ignite a newfound confidence in your ability to live a long, vibrant and joyful life.

— **Shirin Samimi-Fard MD** *Medical Director of Derma Loft, Cologne, Germany*

Return to Beautiful is an outstanding read! It opens your eyes to the things we often put last, ourselves! The book is robust in the areas of optimism, creativity, and confidence. As we age we do need to revolutionize our mindset for ourselves, to be happy, blissful and at peace. This book really opens your eyes to these concepts. Jelena is an outstanding practitioner with extensive training, and it certainly is displayed in *Return to Beautiful*.

— **Dr. Richard Samperisi** *Chiropractic Physician*

Jelena Petkovic has the step by step guide to create beauty from the inside out.

— James Maskell   Founder and CEO Evolution of Medicine and creator of Functional Forum, the world's largest integrative medicine conference

---

Health is the most important asset we have. Many of us struggle on how to get and stay well. In *Return to Beautiful* by Jelena Ley Petkovic, she guides you step by step on how to achieve your health potential. She makes it easy and practical. This is a book everyone should read!

— **Dr. Fab Mancini**   *International bestselling author, speaker and media personality*

Return to Beautiful is a comprehensive approach to helping women feel younger, more energetic and more vibrant. Who DOESN'T need that? Exactly. I was pleased to find that the book offers a very complete method to jumpstart my body and mind to a more healthy and resilient state, with elements of spiritual activation, which I really appreciated. I'll be practicing what I learned here for years to come.

— **Michelle Villalobos**   Personal Brand Strategist, Professional Speaker & Corporate Trainer, Founder of The Women's Success Summit

---

Return to Beautiful

A Journey into Healing,
Flourishing Health and Bliss

Jelena Petkovic PAC MMS

RETURN TO BEAUTIFUL
A Journey into Healing, Flourishing Health and Bliss

ISBN: 978-0-9981728-0-4

Library of Congress Control Number: 2016917445

Cover Design by Nathaniel Dasco.

The publisher has strived to be as accurate and complete as possible in the creation of this book.

The ideas, procedures, and suggestions in this book are not intended as a substitute for the medical advice of your trained health professional. All matters regarding your health require medical supervision. Consult your physician before adapting the suggestions in this book, as well as about any condition that may require diagnosis or medical attention. The author and publisher disclaim any liability arising directly or indirectly from the use of information in this book.

In practical advice books, as in anything else in life, there are no guarantees of health and wellness outcomes. Readers are cautioned to rely on their own judgment about their individual circumstances and to act accordingly.

While all attempts have been made to verify information provided for this publication, the publisher assumes no responsibility for errors, omissions, or contrary interpretation of the subject matter herein. Any perceived slights of specific persons, peoples, or organizations are unintended.

Limit of Liability/Disclaimer of Warranty: The publisher and author make no representations or warranties with respect to the accuracy and completeness of the contents of this work and specifically disclaim all warranties, including without limitation warrantees of fitness for a particular purpose. No warranty may be created or extended by sales or promotional materials. The advice and strategies contained herein may not be suitable for every situation. This work is sold with the understanding that the publisher is not engaged in rendering medical, legal, or other professional advice or services. If professional assistance is required, the services of a competent professional should be sought. Neither the publisher nor the author shall be liable for damages arising therefrom. The fact that an individual, organization or website is referred to in this work as a citation and/or potential resource of further information does not mean that the author or the publisher endorse the information the individual, organization or website may provide or recommendations they/it may make. Further, readers should be aware that web sites listed in this work may have changed or disappeared between when this work was written and when it is read.

SPECIAL GIFT

from Jelena Petkovic

Now that you have your copy of *Return to Beautiful: Journey into Healing, Flourishing Health and Bliss*, you are on your way to creating a life abundant in health, flow and confidence! I'm so excited to share this journey with you, and I know you will continue to not only elevate your life but serve humanity, the planet and all its creatures with a newfound vitality and skill set!

There's so much confusing information out there about healing both our bodies and spirits. I'm ecstatic to provide you with the most effective integrative methods needed to help you heal, reset and activate your life to the one you were destined to lead!

I have created a special bonus to add to your health toolkit, a new meditation basics video. It will help you establish a regular stress management routine and allow you to access your intuition and creativity with more ease. While this video will be offered for sale to the public, you can claim it for free here:

http://ReturnToBeautiful.com/Gift

The sooner you understand the *Return to Beautiful* strategy, the faster you can begin working on your heart's authentic desires!

I'm in your corner. Let me know if I can help further.

Here's to finding your bliss!

Best,

Jelena Petkovic PAC MMS

Jelena Petkovic PAC MMS

Table of Contents

Foreword

I dedicate this book all the teachers before me. To my mentors, whether they knew it or not... Deepak Chopra, Gabrielle Bernstein, Dr. James Gordon, Dr. John Demartini, Dr. Wayne Dyer, the multitude of physicians who set the transformational pace at the Institute of Functional Medicine, and the healers across the globe who have impacted my heart and vision along the way. I have learned so much not only from their knowledge but from their humility, dedication to self-help, and passion for healing and sharing their light.

I also want to give special recognition to those teachers who helped me expand as a human being, the most important ones being my three little children, Valeria, Luka and Mateo. They are the most beautiful lights in my life. Through their eyes and their very being, they have shown me how precious and radiant life is and how much we must live and fight for. I have always felt that children were here to teach us rather than we teach them, and now, by having my own, I have come to know this as a fact. Children are more aligned with the divine energies than most of us may ever come to be as adults. It is important that we listen to them, respect them, and take special care to protect their spirit.

I want to give another special thank you to my parents and the father of my children. Without you I would have never had a chance to grow into the person I have become. You provided me with the foundation of all my growth and exploration. There is no one who could have done this better than you and I will be forever grateful.

Finally, thank you to my grandparents, and all my ancestors who have come before me. You have survived wars, fought hunger, and experienced more hardship than any living being should ever endure. You have struggled through the most trying moments of human evolution and I am eternally grateful. I have your strength and love in my heart and will never forget what you sacrificed and how you suffered so I can have this life.

Blessings, Sat Nam, and Wahe Guru.

Introduction

I remember myself as a toddler. I saw beauty in everything. I was courageous, confident, wild, curious, and positive, and although I depended on my parents for everything, I felt free! I was also healthy, vibrant, abundant, and a magnet of love, encompassing all the elements of whole life wellness. Soon after, however, life, society, and conditioning began and I developed doubt, fear, limiting beliefs, and low self-esteem. Essentially, at a very young age, I had already started to lose the beauty. It was no one's fault that I forgot who I was. I forgot because no one taught me because no one taught them. I had a feeling something was wrong but it took years of failure, searching, learning, and spiritual work to begin to understand what had happened. I spent years trying to figure out how to get back to that confident and radiant toddler, that bliss and that radiant state of health.

Today I will share with you how I found my way home.

Thank you for embarking on this journey. I believe you will heal, you will find flourishing health, and you will be on your way to bliss. I also believe you will discover how absolutely beautiful you are and always were... how beautiful life is and how much mind-blowing beauty there is in all... the good, the bad, the glory, and the failures... and I know you too will find your inner healer, teacher, and leader. I pray this book ignites your inner light and encourages you to believe that by creating more beauty in your life, you hold the key to optimal health. Health should be blissful and it should not be confusing. I believe it's time that, instead of focusing so much effort on teaching toddlers, we help them not to forget how perfectly spectacular they are.

This would be my prescription to the world.

The Beautiful Truth

We are born perfect. Our visions of the world are as beautiful as our physical bodies. We are radiant, plump, awake, lively, energetic, strong and colorful. Our minds match the magnificence of the sky. The whole world seems bright, and we as a part of it are blissful. The fact is that our capacity to maintain this radiance does not decrease as we age, but we somehow forget to see the beauty as we did before and therefore we are more reluctant to create it, to allow it to penetrate us, and therefore our capacity to radiate it also declines.

As we age we encounter fear, toxins, and suffering from our environment. Since no one shows us how to protect ourselves from this suffering, we accumulate it as inflammation and burden in our bodies. This build-up dampens our ability to use our higher brain functions, which is where our capacity to detect and create beauty resides. We are left with a more primitive and limited physiological system, which makes it harder to love ourselves, feed ourselves, or nourish ourselves, let alone try to raise the level of our consciousness to a state that permits bliss.

As babies, we find it easy to find love, and we find beauty in everything. We are trusting and curious. When we need love, we ask for it. We aim to create beauty in all we encounter. We are fascinated with life. We don't question what we deserve or what we need; we demand it, and we take it. When we hear ugly words, we don't believe they are real, and we adjust our perceptions to heal ourselves quickly. We believe everyone loves us and life is good, beautiful and full of adventure.

The resilience we have as babies stems from the fact that we believe everything will be available to us as we need it and that we will not suffer. We have no history of disappointment or failure, and we see hardships as challenges we will get through. We believe that if we are injured, we will heal, and we trust that those around us will give us all we need to make sure we do it quickly.

If we could remain this emotionally, mentally and spiritually fit, our physical being would decline at the slowest rate possible. ***Emotional fitness influences the function of the body***. We would be able to avoid with much more ease that which is not beautiful and, more importantly, toxic to us. We would be able to identify what nourishes our best and healthiest selves. We would choose beautiful and nourishing people, habits, experiences, lifestyles and products because we would see how much more clearly they aligned with who we *really* are. We would confidently be able to take on challenges that bring us closer to our dreams, visions, passions and purposes. We would act in alignment with our true selves, not in alignment with our fear- or ego-based selves. We would regret less, live more, love more, and suffer less from all types of ailments. We would age gracefully, taking with us only wisdom and strength, and have the ability to create, love, inspire and dream to the time of our transition from this earth.

What if we never forgot about how beautiful we are and how beautiful life is? What if we maintained this sense of flow in our lives and made it a habit to cherish our very existence? The only way to raise global vibration, vitality and health is to change the state of conscious awareness in the world and to share these life-enhancing skills with our children. To do this we must start with ourselves as we are today. We must work to see, feel and radiate our purest selves, the most loving, compassionate, curious, hopeful, determined, and resilient version of ourselves, to protect ourselves from disease and to fuel thriving health. We must strategically wake up, clean up, and infuse our mind, body, and spirit with a sense of magnificence so that we know we are worth it, and vital in changing this world to one of more peace and joy.

By now, most of you know that to be healthy you must have a balanced vitality of the mind, body, and spirit. That said, most of us have struggled to understand how this can be done. There are many promises of health... wonder medications, super foods, supplements, fitness practices, yoga, brain training programs, diets, treatments and ways of life. Yet it all seems so overwhelming and most often not sustainable or enjoyable. We start to believe being healthy is painful and difficult. We start to dread health as a thief of our *joy*.

It is sad that, as people age, they find less and less motivation to remain faithful to themselves. They start to "sacrifice" themselves for mainstream beliefs that being unhappy is virtuous. I hear from many patients the common phrases "I have to" or "I need to" do x or y and therefore "I can't take care of myself the way I need to be my most powerful and healthy self." It seems that only those who sell themselves as public icons (models, actors, public office, CEOs) think they are worthy enough to give themselves what they need to function at their optimal level.

The fact is this: maintaining health in modern society is difficult. We now have more chemicals, poorer quality food, less time for leisure, and more stress than ever. This is why chronic diseases (diabetes, cardiovascular disease, autoimmune disease, cancer) are skyrocketing. We are taking more medications than ever and are sicker than ever. We are living longer but look drained, have body pains, and are spreading toxicity with our negative outlook on life. We are depending on others for happiness and for health improvement instead of taking life into our own hands. We are teaching our children that money and success are the most important commodities and that the only way to get them is to sacrifice our very wellbeing.

It is all silly and devastating. The moment has arrived to wake up the beautiful in our lives once more. Enough is enough. There is a way to live a blissful life and live in perfect health. The process I have uncovered is holistic and requires a strategy. Let's let go of depending on doctors, specialists, and experts to diagnose and "fix" you. These healers play a vital role in providing you with education and some guidance, but the real healing depends on *you*. It's time to rediscover your beauty, your instinctive intelligence and confidence. It is time you learn to lead yourself through an experience of self-discovery and commit to yourself.

In this book, I share with you such a journey. It's true this may not be the only journey but it is one that, based on my experience, works. I have collected wisdom from global teachers and merged them to provide people just like you a way back to freedom, healing, and bliss.

The Return to Beautiful process is one that aims to help you build awareness around your body, your mind, and your spirit. The book aims to guide you through an educational experience that will help you understand who you are and what you need to keep yourself safe but expanding toward your true potential.

Staying healthy is a constant journey, and as we age it takes sophisticated processes to keep us feeling and looking fresh so we can continue to spread the love and healing optimism in this increasingly health-challenging environment.

In this book, I will teach you a three-phase holistic strategy to bring back and maintain whole life fitness in your life. Get ready to see, feel, and radiate all the beautiful life has to bring.

Part One

Preparing for the Healing Journey

Don't

Do It, Say It, *or* Think It

Unless It's

Healing,
Loving,
or Beautiful

Chapter 1

Where Are You Now?
Accessing Your Health

Are you struggling through life? Do you have ups and downs and most often confusion on how to keep it all together? Do you reward yourself for the misery by overeating, drinking, complaining or gossiping? If so…you are among the majority! I too was living like this. It was only after a traumatic event in my life that *I woke up*!

I didn't trust myself, or the universe, to take care of me. I pushed and screamed my way toward a life I thought was best for me. I was taught as a child that this is how we got through life because life was HARD! I was taught that life was to be feared and suffering was virtuous.

Because of this, I questioned my every need and desire and was embarrassed when I wanted something that wasn't what I *should* want. I lived not according to my own values but according to those of other people and society. I limited myself because I didn't respect my own soul, instead focusing on pleasing others and living up to society's standards. This of course was an impossible feat. Deep down we all know that if we don't maintain our authenticity and take care of our own health and heart, we will never feel empowered, respected or abundant. The inevitable was that I was left feeling depleted, unsatisfied and uncared for. I didn't feel I had much intrinsic worth and because of that I felt very unstable and even suicidal over any criticism or hint of failure.

Furthermore, I hated myself for not being happy with the "safe life" I had created. This resulted in many years of frustration, confusion, extreme lifestyle habits, anger, low self-esteem, digestive issues, insomnia, and a pregnancy that almost cost me my first child's and my life.

It wasn't until I almost lost my baby girl that I decided to take control over my life. The day I "woke up" was a day I will never forget. It was the last day I ever sat as the victim in my own life. I remember sitting outside of the neonatal intensive care unit, still in my wheelchair after giving birth.

The doctor explained to my husband and babies at the time, the prognosis of my little 900-gram (less than 2 lb.) baby girl. The doctor explained the process of care, the possibilities, and the "reality" of our situation. She also told me to "go home and rest" and not to worry about "doing anything." She told me that medical intervention was best and that not even my breast milk was vital in her care.

I remember feeling more violated, helpless, robbed, guilty, and in more pain than ever before in my life. I thought about suicide as I couldn't fathom being able to deal with what was to come. But suddenly, everything changed. I remembered my strength and my purpose. I remembered my face as a baby. I remembered my passion for healing the world, my love for Mother Teresa, my admiration for Gandhi, and stories of the miracles of John of God. Hadn't I always known inside that I was a healer? Was this not what my whole life had prepared me for? Was this not my redemption for all I had previously not been able to face up to? Was this the ultimate test and therefore my ticket to a new life? I decided to refuse to believe the stories of the darkness and committed to my story of the light. I decided to make this the story that would unveil my true self, not only to myself and my God but to all those who I felt never believed in me. This story would be the one that would transform all my sadness and pain into love. My little girl saved my life. She was the angel who was sent to remind me I had potential to do great things.

After decades of inner drama and turmoil, this day I committed to being the hero of my own life. It was the last day I ever thought of suicide. I decided to start trusting myself, to stop giving so much attention to others' opinions, to nourish myself first and foremost, to enjoy the small pleasures without looking for further reward, to aim for nothing but beauty in every day. I am happy to say I was never the same. I started to question everything and stayed committed to self-compassion and following my heart. I heard the call and, because I never wanted to return to where I came from, I followed the call with conviction.

Of course, it took me another few years of self-improvement and self-love, and a successful twin pregnancy, to get myself to where I felt I truly was the master of my own destiny. During those years, I decided to break all rules that were not mine. I decided to challenge myself to be the person I always wanted to become and to ask myself the hard questions. I decided I deserved to eat the best food; I deserved to take care of my physical, mental, and spiritual health and to strive for greatness. I decided that life was about discovering me, discovering my potential, and then maximizing on all I have learned and acquired for the sake of all sacred and beautiful. I decided I wanted no shortcuts.

How do I hope my story serves you? You may have already had your own "wake up experience" or you may be stuck and wondering how to get to the point at which you are so driven to change and improve. Regardless of why you are reading my words right now, I know you know that there is a better way to live. I know you know that there must be a way to ignite your more beautiful and meaningful life. I know you feel deeply grateful for the life you have been given and feel you want to give more to those you love and possibly serve the world in a bigger way. I'm here to tell you that in this book, there is a way. The "Return to Beautiful" experience is one that strategically makes space for more self-exploration, helping you get physical, mental and emotional blocks out of the way so you can see yourself and your life more creatively. I challenge you to commit to this healing experience. Learn about yourself, what nourishes you, what surprises you, what brings you the most joy. I also ask you to not simply notice things about yourself, but ask yourself *why*. Why do you love it? Why is it so challenging?

The learning in this process is just as important as the transformation. It will provide you with the key to long-term health and wellness and help prevent you from making the same mistakes repeatedly.

If you know watching TV late night triggers your nighttime ice cream binge, it's time to avoid the TV like a plague. If this seems like an unbearable feat, ask yourself why you need to watch TV at night. Can you not sleep? Are you lonely? Is it a way for you to feel connected to the world? Is this your only source of fun?

Any answer might require you to face your issues and resolve them with healthier and equally enjoyable solutions. You need to give yourself what you need so you can live a long, healthy, vibrant life, helping, healing and inspiring others. The world needs you and it's time to take your place among the blissful.

Those who know how to prepare their bodies for best communicating with their true selves are their own best doctors. They can use higher brain functions, live in higher consciousness, and follow intuition. They also can sharpen their senses – feeling, seeing, tasting and listening their way to healing, health, and synchronicity with the divine beauty of the universe.

The importance of the experience lies in the degree of empowerment you achieve from completing it. You will be liberated from all the most common barriers to health – poor diet, lifestyle, chemicals – and instead nourish yourself with vital love, vitamins, and stress-relieving activities.

This liberation and nourishment will give you the vitality and creativity to focus on taking your life to the next level... the level where the magic happens... where you feel in control of your body and mind and can take yourself to a place where you are a magnet for all your heart desires.

Jelena Petkovic PAC MMS

Chapter 2

Staying Healthy in a Toxic World

As I mentioned previously, the modern world in which we live is not supportive of optimal health. We move, rest, and enjoy life too little. We eat too much under-nourishing food. Toxins and chemicals interrupt, bombard, and accumulate in us. These poisons act as hormones and cause inflammation.

Additionally, we hold ourselves to outrageous standards. We multitask and we work long hours and then expect to be great friends, spouses, significant others, and parents. This hazardous living is overloading the body with all types of stress, leading to damaging inflammation and forming more free radicals than the body can ever safely remove and neutralize.

The result is a prematurely aging body, working at sub-optimal levels as it's depleted of nutrients necessary to repair even normal wear and tear. Premature aging is not a mere issue of wrinkles and losing hair. It's a degeneration of all the tissues and healthy physiological processes as they lack the environment to be optimally protected and repaired.

A stressed and inflamed body is one which has poor and inelastic vessels, making them more susceptible to damage and plaque formation, putting you at risk for cardiovascular disease. This body also has overly stressed endocrine glands, leading to deregulation of stress, thyroid and sex hormones. Hormone imbalance leads to a whole host of problems, including poor sugar control and diabetes, infertility, acne, chronic fatigue, and all other related disorders. Finally, the inflammation caused by chemicals, pesticides and other forms of stress lead to major digestive issues, poor nutrient absorption, autoimmune disorders, and gut-brain disorders, further adding to the body's oxidative burden.

So are we doomed to degenerate at accelerated rates while living in our modern toxic wasteland? The answer is definitely not. There is a way to reverse some of the body's damage and prevent further abuse. It's impossible to avoid all toxins, as it's difficult to control things outside of ourselves. What we can do is learn how to limit our exposure to that which is poisonous to our wellbeing and surround ourselves with that which strengthens and nourishes us.

We need to become aware of situations, habits, people, products, and foods that make it very difficult to function. We then need to concentrate on filling up our lives with that which enhances our quality of living, nourishes our body and soul, and helps accelerate us toward the vitality and being we know we can be.

A point I want to highlight right now is that the toxins most harmful to our health are not necessarily physical in nature. Our physical bodies are in fact an accumulation of both experiences and the environment. We are constantly feeding ourselves with sounds, smells, visions, chemicals, nutrients, activities and perceptions that impact how our body functions. Negative perception stimulates stressors such as inflammatory processes in our body, which impact how well we utilize nutrients, produce energy, repair ourselves, and remove toxins.

Our physical body affects how the energy flows through our body as well. If we are inflamed, stiff in certain areas, or weakly built in others, our nervous system cannot flow and send out appropriate chemical messengers to keep us in balance. These chemical messengers are key to managing our digestion, our mood, our hormone systems, our blood sugar and hunger, our immune system, and pretty much every regulating system in our body.

Emotions trigger and release different chemicals to prepare our body for necessary actions. In general, negative emotions often trigger emergency chemical messengers to prepare our body for escape or a fight. Positive emotions trigger relaxing and healing chemical messengers, promoting activities to build, repair and nourish.

These concepts may seem generic right now, but specific strategies for dealing with both external toxins and internal emotional states will be clarified later in this book.

Chapter 3

Understanding the Role of Stress in Aging and Health

Physiological stress is one of the biggest toxins. It is the trigger to a whole host of inflammatory reactions that ultimately impair optimal digestion, repair, mood, energy, and brain function. The trick to controlling stress's impact on our health is to identify when it is occurring, cultivating awareness around both what causes you to be stressed and where in your body you feel stressed. Once you witness the stress occurring, you can then consciously transform the sympathetic response to a parasympathetic response.

The Sympathetic Nervous System (SNS) triggers our "fight or flight response" when we feel threatened. The SNS response is one that we obviously needed in more environmentally dangerous times. During these paleo years, the human body was safer in fear mode, assuming danger rather than safety, and being ready to respond quickly to threats such as wild animals.

The problem with this fast-acting SNS mode is that it streamlines all the body's energy into the emergency systems, nourishing only the larger muscles, the eyes, and the low brain for an efficient self-protective reaction. The Parasympathetic Nervous System (PNS), the "rest and digest" system is either shut down or ignored.

If we spend too much time in SNS mode and neglect PNS mode, over time our bodies start to suffer the consequences. In a non-threatening environment, the PNS is the key to flourishing health. The PNS works to provide nourishment to systems needed to protect, repair, digest and procreate. The PNS is vital for those wishing to live long lives and flourish, as it promotes healthy digestive and metabolic processes, higher brain functions, critical thinking and creativity, and reproductive and hormonal processes.

The real issues start to arise in states of chronic "perceived stress." In chronic perceived stress, people become sensitive to pressures and irritations that are not necessarily dangerous but threaten comfort, rest, organization, concept of self and values. People send out inflammatory messengers and hormones in response to these perceived stressors and find themselves in SNS mode more often than they can recuperate in PNS mode.

The SNS hormones include epinephrine, norepinephrine, cortisol and DHEA. The immediate physiological responses include increased breathing, increased/diverted blood flow to large muscles, dilated pupils, increased arterial blood pressure, increased blood sugar, and increased heart rate. These stress hormones' effects may be harmless in the short term, especially if the perceived stress requires some sort of increased physical activity, but in the long term they wear down the body.

The emotional component associated with stress drains the body's repair and regenerative resources and leave it susceptible to premature aging. Stress in the body translates to increased demand for nutrients that normally act as vital cofactors in immunity, repair, hormone, and detoxification pathways. Stress robs the "unimportant tissues" such as the skin and hair, making poor physical appearance one of the first signs of stress.

More importantly, chronic stimulation of the SNS, stress hormones, and inflammatory signals puts the body at higher risk for disease and shortened life span. The stress response ultimately impacts the body via fatigue, weight gain, cardiovascular stress, glucose intolerance, insulin resistance, and poor pregnancy outcomes. Although poor diets, infection, medications and toxins also place additional burdens on the body, thereby contributing to chronic disease, perceived stress is something we can work to protect ourselves from no matter what our situation is.

What can you do about getting out of stress and into the flow of healthy life? You must start with a plan/strategy for getting back to your *best* self... the self you knew before all the fear and the stress kicked in.

The first part, as mentioned above, involves some self-reflection. "How do I know when stress is taking over? Where do I feel it in my body?" Is it a pain in your neck? Your throat? Your stomach? Is it that you make poor food choices? That you are moody, angry, or mean? Is it that you can't sleep? Is it that you become antisocial? Knowing the signs of when you are suffering from stress overload is the most essential portion of your self-awareness and self-healing. You need to know when it's time to apply a tool.

As I lead you through the Return to Beautiful experience, I will offer you tools such as meditation, mindfulness, breathing, music, and spiritual anchoring to help you transition from SNS "fight or flight" to PNS "repair, digest, repair and procreate" mode.

Some of you will love *all* the tools, while others will find only a few truly nourishing. The important thing is that whatever you discover about yourself, you accept and love unapologetically and unconditionally. Give yourself what you need so that you can live healthy, in bliss and with free energy to shine upon others. We need you to shine. There is no one else who has your unique gifts, passions and love to serve the world. Please don't forget... for the sake of us all!

Chapter 4

Who You Are *and* Why It Matters

As stated before, getting centered on your journey requires you to do some self-exploration. Understanding who you are, your strengths and your passions, can help shift your mindset to one where fear, anxiety, hopelessness, and confusion melt away and your body signals itself to reduce its stress greatly, allowing the body's function to be modulated by the PNS. Functioning from this state of calm and relaxation allows higher brain function and creativity to occur, prevents stress-related inflammation from inducing disease, and allows ideal nutrient absorption, toxin removal, sexual function, and brain nourishment to occur.

The discovery of your spiritual identity can be one of the most healing and joyous feats you have ever attempted. As a teacher of Deepak Chopra's tools of higher consciousness, I ask myself daily "Who am I?" Asking yourself this question every morning can help you:

- Tap into who you are, the self minus the fear, stress, and memories of "shoulds" and "coulds"
- Infuse you with the confidence you need to invest in yourself
- Make your mission a priority, and make you realize that you are, **not** the body you experience this with but the underlying energy that you were born with

Who you are is what you are intuitively drawn to… what you love, how you make others smile, what you do when you have no limitations, how you were when you were two years old and no one told you what you could or couldn't do yet!

Do you know that person? If not, it's time to start exploring!

Here are some questions to get you thinking today. I suggest asking yourself the first three daily, and just watching as your mind unleashes important information for your long-term wellbeing.

- Who am I?
- What do I really, really want?
- What is my purpose?
- What are my strengths?
- How will I use my strengths to serve humanity and the world?
- How has my life prepared me for what I was truly put on the earth to do?
- In an ideal, non-limiting world, what lifestyle nourishes my best self?
- What is my best sleep schedule? Work schedule? Food schedule? Diet? Company?
- What am I truly, truly grateful for?
- What habits, people, and environments stop me from being my best self?
- What legacy do I want to leave behind when I leave this world?
- What is the most important thing for me in my life?

What's my answer? When I ask myself these questions, these come to mind:

- I Am Love
- A Child of The Divine
- A Healer
- A Nurturer of Children
- A Teacher
- A Creative Force
- A Light

If you like any of these, please feel free to connect with them and own them. I believe we are all one and therefore want the same thing… to love, to heal, to teach, and to expand to bliss.

Now it's your turn. Who are you?

_____

_____

_____

_____

_____

_____

_____

Test yourself and answer the "I am" question daily. See what stays consistent as you repeatedly ask and listen as you receive the answer to this soul-deep question.

A Tip on Making Self Discovery Fun

Use Pinterest to make a series of vision boards. Grab pictures and words that match your essence.

I love using Pinterest as my early evening pick-me-up activity. It takes just 5-10 minutes and can help you organize your ideas about who you are. Pick pictures, quotes and mantras that you are attracted to… not that you "should want" or "should have." Stay away from judgment and just pick the pictures you love. Start four pages showing 1) my body 2) my energy 3) my purpose 4) my life.

Chapter 5

Spiritual Empowerment for Flourishing

Spirituality is not necessarily derived from religion. It is simply what gives people a deep sense of meaning and the ability to overcome challenges and crises with more ease. Spirituality can be anything that gives you higher purpose or meaning, from being part of nature to pride in overcoming a difficult illness or life-threatening event. Spiritual beliefs are strongly connected with your community, activities that bring you peace, the things that bring you strength, the things you care about, the things that excite you, and the things most important to your wellbeing.

There are close to 300 evidence-based studies that link degree of health to degree of spirituality. Those who consider themselves to be more spiritual have been shown to have lower blood pressure, sleep better, be more satisfied in life, have more energy, have better mental health, and have lower overall mortality when faced with illness.

It wasn't until my late 20s that I began my own spiritual re-awakening. That's when I gave birth to my first child, my daughter, Mila Valeria. She was born very prematurely and weighed under 2 lbs. I knew that my spiritual misalignment and subsequent nervous and anxious demeanor had much to do with her traumatic early arrival.

This mini-preemie was faced with a whole host of medical challenges and a poor prognosis. I decided at that moment that I would no longer fight my divine connection and my power to completely change my destiny. I would not allow the lies I told myself, or was told by others, to impact my wellbeing any longer. I decided to commit to both the healing of myself and her recovery and health. I decided to ignore the statistics presented to me and instead went within and vowed to facilitate a series of miracles.

I meditated and prayed 8+ hours a day as I pumped my milk and gathered all positive healing light and energy from all corners of the earth to envision the healing of every cell of her body. I watched as this little girl fought and jumped every hurdle. I thanked every tube, doctor, and drop of milk as it healed my daughter. I said a silent thank you up to 1000 times a day. With every inhalation, I channeled my divine self and with every exhalation I breathed this love into my daughter and everyone who prayed or played a role in her healing.

I believe it was because of all this that my daughter beat all the odds. Today she is one of the most vibrant and healthy 7-year-olds I know. This experience taught me that healing and medicine came from a much deeper plane than anyone had ever spoken to me about.

I began to research the nervous system, and the impact of stress and inflammation on health, exploring and taking courses in eastern medical modalities, such as acupuncture, meditation, yoga, and shiatsu as sources of understanding. I embarked on a journey into the realm of eastern medicine. I studied to be a yoga teacher, a shiatsu healer, and even pondered going back to school as an eastern medicine practitioner.

It wasn't until after I had my healthy twin boys in 2011 that I decided I wanted to radically improve my quality of being. Ultimately, I decided not to abandon my traditional western medicine education. Instead, I expanded and integrated mind-body medicine, functional medicine, Ayurveda lifestyle medicine, and spiritual healing practices into the way I care for patients.

More importantly, I found that as I dug deeper into the origins of health I began to revisit my relationship with a higher source. I decided to serve patients with the help of the spiritual connection I was cultivating, allowing myself to speak from a place of experience, intuition, love and compassion with the people I wanted to help.

Because of this, I feel that I do more good today as a life guide than a medical practitioner, allowing patients to discover on their own what serves and nourishes them, empowering them with my faith in them and the miracles they can create with commitment to and within themselves.

Spirituality, in my opinion, is the vessel for the most profound healing and life experiences.

So... How can we all get a bit more spiritual?

- **Connect with nature.** Nature gives us the sense of knowing that there is something much bigger than ourselves guiding us, fueling us and watching over us.

- **Pray.** Ask for guidance, strength, ability to connect, ability to listen, ability to know. Ask whatever you feel is your divine source: god, love, the universe, your higher self.

- **Repeat mantras of devotion and love.** These allow you to melt fear, and connect with the most beautiful part of you, the true part, the one most aligned with your intuition and divine source. Nothing does this better for me than Kundalini Yoga. Mantra songs (shared later in the book) can help you effectively connect with your higher self, transcend ego, fear and negativity, and act from a place of pure love. If you need a quick start, go to my Jelena Petkovic Spotify List, follow me and find a few playlists dedicated to Kundalini mantras there.

- **Meditate.** Meditation allows you to remove the ego of the present and the karma of the past. Over time it will clear your mind of false perceptions and beliefs about who you are and what is real, allowing you to have more flexibility, curiosity, compassion, and peace in your life, ultimately living with less anxiety and more flow.

- **Give gratitude.** Giving gratitude is a fast track to love and to health, taking away inflammation associated with anger, regret, and pain, which will help you create a more harmonious inner environment.

- **Take care of yourself in a way in which you can act for your greatest good.** By acknowledging our strength and values, we give ourselves and others a mindful perspective, allowing more compassion and flow as we work to optimize the world using our gifts. Too often we push ourselves, or others, to be something we are not. This results in pushing ourselves to live in a certain way and believe certain things that are against our very core. This misalignment creates distress, unhappiness and inability to see the beauty all around us. For this reason we must remove from our lives the removable things that cause us stress, we must nourish ourselves with things that bring us health, and we must seek to build on what we most naturally want to share with the world.

Chapter 6

Using Mantras to Help Manifest Bliss

A mantra is an instrument or vehicle of the mind. It can help you expand beyond your limited perception of the world or yourself into a being of endless possibilities. I use mantras to fight my own blocks to health, happiness and success.

To pick a mantra, you should first be aware of what your limiting beliefs are. Is it that you don't think you're worth it? Is it that you think there is something wrong with your health or because you have some condition that makes you feel less whole? Is it that you feel you're not special enough? Is it that you don't love yourself enough? Is it that you don't feel radiant? Is it that you worry too much? Is it that you don't trust yourself?

List 3 limiting beliefs you will actively work on in the next six (6) weeks.

1._____

2._____

3._____

There are many mantras used to help unblock all types of fears, doubts and mind blocks. Below, I list a few of my favorites.

Try saying your mantra(s) 40 times while brushing your teeth every day in the mirror, or writing one down on a piece of paper 40 times while on a brain break at work. Watch your mindset shift.

- I Am Enough.
- I Am Healthy, Happy, Whole.
- I Am Light and Live to Shine.
- I Am Giving, Loving and Abundant.
- I Am Playful, I Am Powerful, I Am Compassionate, I Am of the Divine.
- I Am Beautiful and Blissful.
- I Dedicate Each Day to My Enlightenment.
- I Am Perfect and Will Use My Intuitive Intelligence to Heal Myself and the World.

Chapter 7

The Utlimate Diet... Eat Like You Love Yourself

Food choices and eating habits make a big impact on your overall wellbeing. According to Ayurvedic medicine philosophies (more on this Chapter 26), and Hippocrates, food can be your best medicine, but it can also be your biggest barrier to flourishing health.

According to the Institute of Functional Medicine, food is both information and connection. Our genes cannot be coded if they do not have the right nutrients to express their traits favorably. Because of this our genes *do not* identify us; we are simply an expression of the way they are impacted by their environment.

Food is one of the most important environmental influencers and, therefore, we are at the mercy of the food we feed ourselves. Nutritious food can maximize our genetic potential, while other food choices can bring out all of our genetic vulnerabilities.

Food also connects us to certain types of relationships. Our diet and our health can be greatly impacted by those we choose to surround ourselves with. We become the diet of our peers, friends and lovers... this is important when making healthy lifestyle changes. We must actively search for those who will support our healthier lifestyle and, therefore, share with us our passion for healthier food.

Now, if removing/avoiding certain people from your life is either impossible or not desired, I recommended a heart-to-heart conversation with them. It's amazing what people will accept when asked kindly. Many of my patients have had to ask those loved ones and friends who felt defensive about any restrictive lifestyle to support them. It is important to explain that it's only for a limited time and that it is very important to you to "stick with the program" as it is an act of self-love that you desire.

Once you explain the reasons and the benefits, they may even want to join you! Furthermore, most who watch you transform into a more confident and vibrant version of you will not need any further explanation. You will inevitably become their inspiration, their health guru, and their motivation.

During each phase of the Return to Beautiful journey, you will be asked to change the way you eat. The diet prescribed helps you reach the mind, body, and spiritual objective of your healing journey.

Phase 1 focuses on helping the body remove barriers to health. Removing foods that cause inflammation and toxicity is key in this phase. Detoxifying the body is not simple. It must be strategic. It depends not only on what you don't eat, but also on what you do eat. Additionally, removing unhelpful eating schedules and habits helps the body process the foods better. You will discover how to align your eating strategy with the natural rhythm of your body and nature, leading to better digestion and metabolic nutrient assimilation for optimal physiologic function. To help you prepare for the nutritional portion of the Return to Beautiful experience, please see The Return to Beautiful Shopping List (Chapter 31 Section A).

Phase 2 focuses on feeding a healthy microbiome (or microbe population) in your body. Most people are not aware of this, but our bodies are more microbes (bacteria, yeast, fungi and bacteria) than cells. In fact, we have ten times more of these microbes than human cells, and these microbes determine our wellbeing. The microbiome controls not only our digestive functions but also our mood, vitality, and health. During Phase 2, we work to feed the "good" population of bacteria while starving out the remaining "bad" population of microbes that persist despite removing their source of nourishment in Phase 1.

The good bacteria are "good" because they help us optimally metabolize our food, get the most nutrients out of whatever we eat, prevent the invasion and circulation of pathogens, and protect us from the toxic effects of accumulating inflammatory and chemical metabolites. Considering their mass prevalence, the microbiome's gene pool is thought to be even more important than our own.

As stated previously, there are approximately ten times more bacteria than cells in our body, and their gene pool is up to 100 times more active in producing proteins that communicate directly with our own human genome, influencing their behavior and regulation. This means that the bacteria living within us could be the deciding factor in which genetic mutations are expressed and which genetic mutations are suppressed, holding the key to our wellbeing.

When we harbor a healthy population of microflora, the proteins produced by their genes help us make sure inflammation and oxidation are kept at bay, and cell signaling, metabolism and detoxification are ideal. A well-functioning metabolism means optimal repair functions; healthier tissues, skin, and nails; and better weight control. Poor microbes in the digestive tract predispose us to a whole host of issues, including inflammatory conditions such as arthritis, autoimmune diseases, blood sugar irregularities, cardiovascular disease, hormone and fertility problems, and mood imbalances.

Phase 3 focuses on energy, longevity, vitality, and superfoods. Now that we have cleaned out the body of barriers to best health in Phase 1, and improved metabolism and digestive health in Phase 2, it's time to focus on preventing premature aging and disease and ultimately activating the tissues so they are proactively creating the most youthful and highly functioning internal environment.

The goal of this phase is to maximize on your genetic potential, which means using food to express your DNA as favorably as possible, continuing to nourish the microbiome, and providing a surplus of protective nutrients for challenged systems. Protocols including certain superfoods, dietary guidelines based on your underlying energy, and life-extending supplements and eating methods will be shared with you in Phase 3.

Phase 3 dietary guidelines are to be used indefinitely until you see reason to revert to Phase 1 again. All three phases will be more fully explained further in the book.

The When and How of Eating

What you eat is important, but so is why and how you eat. Spending a day or two simply observing how your mood, stress level and overall attitude impact your food choices and eating patterns can bring you lots of wisdom. Awareness is key in helping you personalize your healing journey. Managing stress around meals can be a key to long-term health.

Weight management prevents many chronic diseases. With the current obesity epidemic, we need to be more proactive about watching the quality of what and how we eat. Studies have shown that chronic life stress is associated with a greater preference for energy- and nutrient-dense foods high in sugar and fat (Torres & Nowson, et al., 2007).

An essential question for those who find they regret certain meals or food choices is "At what time of day do you make the poorest choices (overeating, eating something you regret, eating too fast)?" Once you can pinpoint a time of day, you might squeeze in a self-care tool around this time. You can carry some healthy fruits and vegetables to eat in case you need them, take a walk, meditate, drink some tea, listen to a song that brings you happiness and love, take a break and work on your vision board, or just practice some deep breathing around this time. Experiment with different practices to help you combat the real reason for overeating.

Another good question is "What situations or emotions trigger eating in a way that is not in alignment with your optimal health vision?" If certain people, situations, or emotional topics trigger certain relationships with food, you need to start naming the behavior as you get triggered, and either work to break up the cause from the effect or get yourself out of "fight or flight" primitive brain mode and into the higher brain functions of "rest and digest." The best solution I have found is to avoid triggers for 2 - 3 weeks as you work on stress reduction. If you can't avoid the trigger, then use one or a few of these in the order they appear: 1) 10 deep breaths, inhaling 5 seconds through your nose and exhaling 5 seconds through your mouth, 2) take a walk and look at the sky, 3) look at one of the pictures you have on Pinterest reminding you of the person you want to become, and 4) drink a tall glass of water.

Chapter 8

Lifestyle, Habits and Your Environment

The habits you create can either challenge or support your overall wellness. Habits that cause stress, inflammation, or pollution of your body obviously make it harder for your body to preserve itself and keep up with the simple repairs associated with daily wear and tear.

The brain has been evolving for over 300 million years. Our experiences and the way we perceive them have impacted the evolution of our genetic behavior and our very biology. Our habits can support or challenge our ability to thrive. The habits you choose today impact your body of tomorrow.

The body is said to replace 98% of its atoms each year. We are constantly changing and, therefore, can actively decide if we wish to be reborn into something stronger and healthier, or if we won't bother to intervene, making us weaker and more susceptible to disease.

Habits of Health

For most, aging brings about challenges that make healthy habits more difficult to keep. As we age we tend to adopt poor habits to manage the stress of life. Most of us find we need instant gratification to make life bearable. It is often this belief that we cannot live in the way that truly speaks to our soul that puts us in danger of addiction and harmful habits.

We believe that we must work 10-hour days to gain respect and money for "grownup things." This leads us to a $2000/year wine habit (and this is just four drinks a week!) or, worse, anxiety or depression (that could cost over $300,000 over a lifetime). For the sake of a bigger house and a car, we don't join a nice gym and we save money on food, putting us at heightened risk of diabetes, heart disease, and other autoimmune diseases (costing over $10,000 per year per patient).

It is when we stop giving our happiness and wellbeing importance that we often develop abusive habits. The idea that life is supposed to be stressful and oppressive saps our creativity and our love of life, and makes healthy habits seem difficult or last priority.

Meanwhile, it is the very act of removing unhelpful habits and adopting rejuvenating ones that can make a difference in how resistant or resilient you are to disease, premature aging, low mood, low energy, and poor decision making.

Some habits, like smoking and drinking, are obviously poor health habits. Others, like watching TV after dinner, staying up late at night, sitting for more than a few hours, depending on alcohol or drugs to bring you joy or rest, eating large/heavy dinners, and sleeping poorly are still practiced by many who don't question the impact these habits have on their health or their ability to flourish.

When my patients come to me for a whole health and life reset, I arrange their day so that their schedule matches their natural circadian rhythms of optimal activity, rest, and metabolism. Furthermore, I incorporate the traditional wisdom of both Ayurveda and traditional Chinese medicine in regards to healthy lifestyle.

According to Deepak Chopra's teachings, the five pillars of wellbeing should be (a) quality sleep, (b) meditation, (c) movement, (d) balanced emotions, and (e) proper nutrition.

According to this intelligence, people should be in bed by 9:30 PM and sleeping by 10 PM to allow full detoxification, immunity, and repair processes to occur. Those who are asleep between 10 PM and 2 AM are much more likely to recover from the day's drama than those who miss out on these key hours of rest.

Other habits that are helpful include waking around 5 AM - 6 AM to meditate 10 - 30 minutes, followed by a stretch and movement before breakfast around 7 AM - 8 AM. Breakfast should be nutritious but not heavy. Green and herbal teas should be sipped between meals to promote satiety and calm, and aid in proper bowel motility and clearing.

Sitting down to enjoy meals, savoring food, and giving gratitude for each morsel or sip can make a big difference in how you utilize the nutrients. Daily gratitude and meditation sessions are key in improving immune function, promoting heart rate variability, and, on a quantum level, send out vibrations to attract more synchronicity in your life, or flow, helping you attract more of what you want in life.

Numerous publications and research now prove that gratitude is a major player in all realms of success including health, business, and social arenas. Research by Robert Emmons and Michael McCullough has shown that those who focus on gratitude have greater emotional and physical health.

Gratitude practices have been shown to cultivate benefits which include (a) more joy and happiness, (b) fewer days ill, (c) regular physical activity, (d) more energy, (e) more determination and focus, (f) better sleep, (g) more optimism, (h) better family relationships, (i) increased strength and resilience to stress, and (j) greater likelihood of serving others.

Making it a habit to take time to see the beauty in everyone and everything daily can help cultivate a state of gratitude, allowing you to value life and yourself more. These practices can also help you bring out the best in people and can help you give and receive more support and love. Searching for and seeing beauty means having faith in love, having faith in yourself, and promoting an ideal environment for peace, healing, flourishing health and bliss.

This said, beauty can be hard to find when you're suffering physically, your digestive health is poor, your lifestyle rhythms are off, or you don't have the right practices, tools and people around you.

Return to Beautiful will help you adopt the five pillars of wellbeing into your life. Once you have these, staying in line with who you are and with your true desires will be much easier. Additionally, you will begin to feel more nourished, creative and empowered to cultivate the ideal environment to radiate, project, and mirror sustainable health of the mind, body, and soul. I believe flourishing can be easy if we reset you back to your best state of being, to the state where beauty is everywhere, and then use tools such as meditation and moment to moment awareness to keep you on your true path.

Environmental Toxins

Our environment can either nourish or challenge our ability to live life to the fullest. Unfortunately for most of us, our day-to-day environment is quite toxic. Modern life has surrounded us with a host of chemicals, pesticides, plastics and other artificial materials that, ultimately, become absorbed and woven into our bodies, challenging our health. As we age, the chemicals we inhale, ingest, and absorb accumulate, placing additional burdens on organs and tissues.

These unwanted pollutants challenge our very ability to function as we should, adding work for the liver, and mimicking the action of certain hormones, throwing off our endocrine pathways. Our body relies heavily on our endocrine system, as these hormones act as signals to keep our body in harmony. Endocrine imbalance can make functions such as weight management, sugar balance, getting pregnant, pleasant mood, growth and repair, metabolism, reducing inflammation, and stress management very difficult.

Additionally, these chemicals and toxins cause oxidative damage, depleting our body of essential antioxidants and aging our bodies at accelerated rates. Pesticides have become especially damaging to our digestive health, causing inflammation and contributing to the chronically debilitating process known as leaky gut, and predisposing us to many inflammation-induced conditions, including autoimmune disease, mood disorders, cancers, diabetes, and heart disease.

Many of these chemicals have been found to disrupt normal hormone function, contributing to many modern-day chronic illnesses such as obesity, low sperm count, male offspring feminization, insulin resistance, diabetes and low birth weight infants (EWG, n.d; Stahlhut et al., 2007; Sun, et al., 2014).

BPA, for example, has been specifically linked to several health concerns (hormone alterations, obesity and cancer among them) and many studies are still pending to tell us the exact repercussions of this chemical's toxicity.

One of the most worrisome associations has been found between chemicals and breast cancer trends. Environmental chemicals are now thought to be related to the rising risk of breast cancer in those with no genetic risk (Breast Cancer Fund, 2013).

Knowing this is happening, what can we do to thrive despite our toxic environments?

1. Know where the toxins are and *avoid* them!
2. Make sure you ingest a surplus of antioxidant rich foods, while occasionally giving your liver extra TLC for a therapeutic detoxification.

Where are the environmental toxins and how do we avoid them?

Pesticides, chemicals, and metals build up in our systems from a multitude of sources. On their own, these impurities can burden the body, but together they challenge our very ability to function normally and accelerate us toward premature aging and chronic disease. Although we cannot avoid toxins altogether, we can minimize their effects by preventing exposure from some of the most direct products we encounter.

Here are some tips to decrease your toxic load.
1. Avoid BPA.

    BPA (Bisphosphenol A) is a carbon-based synthetic chemical compound that is found in plastics and epoxy resins. When absorbed into the body, BPA acts as a hormone, altering natural endocrine behavior in certain concentrations. We are exposed to BPA via cans, plastic bottles, receipts, CDs, DVDs, water pipes and sports equipment.

    Although BPA is almost impossible to avoid altogether, limiting exposure may be important to overall health, preventing certain chronic disease, infertility, and even cancer. More specifically, avoid BPA by:

    - Ask for all receipts to be emailed electronically. Thermal recipes contain traces of the endocrine disruptor known as BPA. A study conducted by the EWG showed that about 40% of all tested receipts tested positive for this chemical. It seems the resin on the thermal paper is the major source of toxicity here.

    - Carry your filtered water in glass or BPA-free water bottles. Invest in a water filter at home, and fill up one or a few bottles before leaving the house for the day.

    - Do not eat canned foods, especially if they don't have the BPA-free label. BPA is found in the aluminum can lining and leaches into your food, accumulating in your body.

- Stop using plastic food storage bags or containers, especially in the freezer or in the microwave, as extreme temperatures accelerate leaching BPA and other endocrine-disrupting chemicals into your foods.

- Choose BPA-free toilet paper. Yes, 80-90% of tested toilet paper showed positive for BPA, per a study reported in the Journal of Environmental Science & Technology. Recycling of paper seems to be the reason why this chemical has gotten into your paper and into your body via your most intimate parts. Since the freshly tree sourced options are most often put through another toxic process, namely bleaching, this option is controversially worse, considering the double health and environmental burden. What to do? The best option seems to be tree-free toilet paper made from sugar cane... or washing! I leave you with this information for you to decide! Awareness is the first step to better and safer options.

2. Avoid common sources of hormones, pesticides, processed sugars, metals and preservatives.
   - Buy organic, locally grown, whole and fresh produce.

   - Consume only grass-fed, hormone free, non-GMO fed and humanely raised animals.

   - Avoid dairy milk with genetically engineered recombinant bovine growth hormone (rBGH or rBST).

- Don't eat processed or prepackaged food which has leached BPA or phthalates from the packaging they sit in.

- Avoid PCBs and mercury-ridden fish by choosing wild fish and using Omega 3 supplements derived from krill oil or wild Alaskan salmon.

- Check your water supply, your bathroom, and your kitchenware to make sure you're not being infected with toxins without knowing it.

- Place reverse osmosis filters in your home for both drinking and bathing. Your skin may be an even more important mechanism for absorbing chemicals, such as hormone disruptors, herbicides, and metals, especially when wet and the pores are dilated for deeper penetration over a large surface area.

- Replace your non-stick pots and pans with ceramic or glass cookware.

- Replace plastic cooking utensils with wood and metal ones.

3. Be *very* picky about what you put on or near your skin.

There are thousands of synthetic chemicals used in our personal care products and cosmetics (Breast Cancer Fund, n.d).

Of the 20% tested for their safety, many have been linked to a variety of health issues, including (a) cancer, (b) developmental issues, and (c) disorders of both a physical and a behavioral nature (The Campaign for Safe Cosmetics, n.d).

Furthermore, these products we put on our face or on our babies are made in factories that use toxic pesticides, cleaners, and grease to keep things "sterile," suggesting the ingredient lists do not account for the full impact the product has on our health (Breast Cancer Fund, n.d).

The Campaign for Safe Cosmetics has reported that 1 in 5 of the products tested contains chemicals linked to cancer and 80% of products have impurities of questionable safety (The Campaign for Safe Cosmetics, n.d; Campaign for Safe Cosmetics, pink ribbon).

Deepening the concern, many products have now added advanced ingredients, devised to help deliver contents of product even deeper into the skin, putting consumers at heightened risk from the ingredients of questionable safety (The Campaign for Safe Cosmetics, n.d).

Since the FDA does not regulate the ingredients of cosmetic and personal care products, it has authorized a Cosmetic Ingredient Review panel (CIR) to oversee chemical groups' safety profiles for human health. Concern lies in the fact that while the European Union has banned over 1000 chemicals from cosmetics, the CIR has banned less than a dozen (EWG, n.d; U.S. Food and Drug Administration, 2000).

Many modern chronic diseases, including breast cancer, are now thought to be influenced by exposure to environmental chemicals. The Breast Cancer Fund is at the forefront of research and awareness, educating all on how avoiding certain environmental chemicals may be key in breast cancer prevention (Breast Cancer Fund, 2013).

Below are the steps to decrease your risk.

1. Replace conventional personal care products with those listed on the EWG Skin Deep website or make your own DYI beauty products. Be especially careful when it comes to products for small children... organic USDA labels and phthalate-, paraben-, silicon-, fragrance- and sulfate-free are a must. More information about clean personal care products and DYI recipes can be found at my site, AntiAgingSavantess.com.

2. Avoid Triclosan. Triclosan is a chemical which acts as an endocrine (hormone) disruptor that decreases our resistance to chemicals and affects our mood, metabolism and overall ability to function optimally. Triclosan is found in hand sanitizers. Look for Triclosan- and alcohol-free for best results.

3. Choose household products, mattresses, and furniture that are free from PBDEs, formaldehyde, antimony, boric acid and brominated chemicals. Choose materials that are naturally less flammable such as leather, wool, cotton and silk. Forget clothing and furniture that says stain- or water-resistant and forget carpets as they contain perfluorinated chemicals (PFCs).

4. Remove toxic dust by routinely using a HEPA vacuum to avoid inhalation of food contamination and skin absorption.

5. Be wary about conventional cleaning supplies. Avoid chemicals such as 2-butoxyethanol (EGBE) and methoxydiglycol (DEGME) that have been linked to infertility and harm to fetuses. Look for greener alternatives. Look for organic, eco-friendly, and non-toxic products.

- Use natural cleaning products or make your own. Baking soda and vinegar are staple ingredients for DIY cleaning.

- Avoid fabric softeners and dryer sheets, which infuse your clothes with toxic fragrances and other chemicals.

6. Replace your plastic shower curtains with fabric curtains.

Now that you know *where* the toxins potentially lie, it's your job to avoid them to the best of your ability. If you don't think you can avoid *all* these products in your everyday life, do as much as you can while leading yourself through the *Return to Beautiful* experience.

We want to decrease the stress on your body as much as possible during this time so we can focus on maximal repair, nourishing and strengthening. The more of a break we can give the body, the more effective our efforts will be and the more transformative the experience.

If all this seems *way* too stressful, I suggest focusing on removing plastic from your life and focus on using as many non-toxic personal care products as you can.

Chapter 9

Relationship Makeover

Do you trust your tribe?

Do they support you?

Do you feel like there are people who drain you?

Is there someone who you feel is toxic?

You must understand that if there is someone especially damaging to your life, they are also damaging to your health.

I'm not saying to be vicious and tell them they do not serve you. I am asking you to gently let them know that you are working on something in your life and will not be as social or communicative with many people while you are working on improving your life. You can also not say anything and just play the "busy" card for the sake of self-preservation.

I ask you to choose your tribe, your friends and those you have a choice to associate with which mirrors the best part of you, inspires you and elevates you. People often mirror to you their own insecurities and fears and can for that reason be quite toxic and damaging to those they project onto.

It's really not their fault... in fact you might have once been in their shoes. Those who act out of fear, hate or toxicity are most probably suffering themselves or on a lower plane of consciousness and are plagued by damaging and narrow beliefs which have shaped their world in such a way that they feel threatened by anyone who doesn't live in alignment with them.

Again, it's not their fault. Show them love, show them light, and protect yourself from them if they still feel too heavy for you to bear.

These people may reenter your life again, when they have expanded or when you are stronger and less affected by their fear.

How to find a better circle.

During your experience, especially the first time around, it's important to find a circle of support. Finding people, you can trust your true self with can be tough. Healthy friendships and support mean they are living with a similar level of awareness and understand that any negativity or fear they have is rooted within and not a reflection of the person they are judging or projecting onto.

For this reason, finding friends who mirror your favorite and most beautiful self is important. It means they have worked on themselves, love themselves, have compassion for themselves, and therefore see only the strengths, love and potential in others. You know you are speaking to a healthy friend when your heart soars when you are with them, when your body seems light, when you can laugh at even the craziest of scenarios, and when they look you in the eye with deep compassion. If you cannot feel these qualities in your friends and companions, they may not be the best support for you at this time of transformation and growth.

Conscientious people can be found anywhere but can be found at higher densities in yoga and meditation studios and spiritual workshops and retreats. I know I've found many like-minded friends at yoga, spiritual meet-up groups, medical conferences aimed at Mind Body Healing, at Deepak Chopra's Center, through Gabrielle Bernstein's Spirit Junkie Master classes, and through Mind Valley Academy's A-Fest. Other events may include Tony Robbins' workshops or the Summit at Sea.

With every person, I've met with this elevated consciousness, I've felt more supported and loved, and because of this I've felt stronger in my efforts to ditch the habits not in alignment with the person I truly was and the person I aimed to become.

Social acceptance and support is not just nice to have; it's essential to wellbeing and long-term health. Lack of social support has been linked to the same health risks as physical inactivity and diabetes; some claim it to be even more hazardous to health than smoking (Yeang, Boen, Gerken, et al. 2016).

So, before you take the leap into transforming your health and life, know that your social network's health will also have to match that of your optimal mind/body/spirit. For those with intimate partners who they love and want to maintain, a plan must be made to get the partner fully informed of your wishes. I advise you sit down and explain to them the need for a healing experience and that it is very important they support your healing and nourishing lifestyle during this time.

Children must also be told the importance of the parent's journey. One explanation could be "Mommy/Daddy needs to eat/live/work/behave/sleep a certain way for a while so that their body can be the strongest, healthiest and most energetic possible. This will help me help you even better than I am now. I want to be the happiest parent for you so that I can make sure you are the happiest child/children. If you want to help me, I can teach you what I am doing and you can keep me company as I take care of myself. Thank you for being a part of my life and my journey to be my best self. I love you."

Making children a part of your healing process can empower them and help build their confidence as a healer and teacher. I tell my children daily that they are the ones who teach and heal me, and that they take care of me as much as I take care of them. I see their faces light up and know they will take that energy back to the world.

The chart below will help you become more aware of the quality of your social network. Do they support you? Figuring out where you may need more support can be a great step toward getting it. Having a conversation with those who have been making health hard for you can also be an opportunity to bring them to awareness about their own state of health.

My one caveat is, when discussing health with others, it's important not to impose your beliefs onto them. Don't try to convince them. Speak to those you want to influence by speaking about what you want and what you are doing or need to do to reach your visions of freedom, flourishing health and bliss! As I mentioned before, once you start to radiate the benefits of this journey, I am confident you will be a natural leader in the realm of health and happiness.

For some inspiration and support, follow me on Instagram (@heartandsoulmedicine) and share your thoughts and comments on my Facebook page (ABeautifulRx by Jelena Petkovic).

Social Network Assessment

Social Network Assessment Form

Social Network	How Supportive	How Unsupportive	Plan
Intimate partnership			
Work			
Immediate family			
Extended family			
Friends			

Chapter 10

Moving You to a Clean and Beautiful Life

If you are trying to lose weight, optimize the way your body functions, and prevent early aging, exercise is a key component. This said, I encourage you to focus on the diet and lifestyle homework first, and then add in the exercise when you are more confident with the diet and schedule.

I find that most of my patients exercise already, and that although exercise is key for long-term health, it is not necessarily the most vital component in this experience. In fact, many of my patients exercise too much! They fight their poor habits and nutrition by overcompensating with exercise and often suffer from fatigue, irritability and chronic inflammation. Too much exercise can cause problems including physiological stress, binge eating, inflammation, poor sleep, and anxiety.

In general, the transformation occurs when you do something completely different than what you are doing in your regular lifestyle. I urge you to adopt as many foreign or new habits and tools as possible during your journey. The adoption of these newer habits will be the real game changers in your health... this is where the magic occurs. Those of you who already work out regularly may benefit more from focusing on rest, nutrition, self-love practices, stress relief, and removing barriers that are polluting your mind, body and spirit.

This said, I have suggested types of exercise that best complement the objective of each phase of the program. Phase 1 is your detoxification phase and sweating will be key in aiding this process. Because of this, I suggest that my patients focus on cardio and Bikram yoga. Daily breathing and stretching are also key to help eliminate unwanted elements from the body.

Phase 2 is the nourishing and repair phase. The exercises suggested during this phase include daily walks, yoga and dance.

Phase 3 is the activation phase. During this phase the exercise routines should be balanced. Cardio, strength-focused training, and yoga should be alternated. This is where you are best suited to challenge your body. Start taking a Boot Camp (Barry's is my favorite), join CrossFit, start a fitness challenge, prepare for a marathon, go on a cycling trip, or climb Mount Everest.

Exercise and Movement

Movement is different than exercise and in my opinion more important. Making movement a habit can be challenging with modern schedules and lots of jobs in front of the computer and on the phone. For this reason, it takes some creativity, strategy and dedication to make sure that we move often and throughout the day.

Studies have shown that sitting more than six hours a day can be detrimental to your health and increase your risk of chronic disease. Some studies have even shown that sitting can be as deadly as cigarettes. Movement has cardiovascular benefits as it tones the heart and keeps the blood and fluid exchange throughput in the vessels optimal. With movement, the digestive system is always getting a massage and gravity can better assist efficient waste removal. Movement alone assists better circulation of lymph fluids so that the immune system can work to remove pathogens and toxins. Additionally, movement works to improve overall mood, and if done in nature it can serve a multitude of health purposes, including lowering stress hormones, pulse rate, and blood pressure, and improving mood and mindfulness (Environmental Health Preventative Medicine, 2010).

In an ideal world, we would move before each meal, then stretch, then do some breathing exercises, give gratitude for our food, and then sit down to eat our meals with gratitude, real need, and grace. Although including these activities in your daily life may seem overwhelming in long run, I ask you to make a special effort during the initial four weeks.

Once your health is revived and reset, your newfound vitality and creativity will naturally make healthy life rhythms easy.

Chapter 11

Meditations and Mindfulness for Sustainable Bliss

To me, meditation is the basis of all health maintenance. Without meditation, life can seem confusing, overwhelming, stressful, frightening, and/or aggressive. The reason for this is that, without appropriate "inner" fitness, your internal environment starts to resemble these very qualities. As we experience life and its numerous challenges, without appropriate tools to metabolize, detoxify, purify and heal ourselves, our perception of what is real is easily manipulated into chaotic disarray.

An analogy would be attempting to drive a car without windshield wipers. Eventually the dirt accumulated along the journey will make the drive quite difficult and dangerous. Like the windows of this wiper-less car, your brain will tend to accumulate spots, clouding its awareness, causing it to use muddled information to make decisions and navigate life. Over time, an unfit mind will skew your perception, and you will project this inaccurate vision onto any person or situation you encounter, mirroring your internal disarray onto your understanding of the outside world and into your relationships.

Meditation and mindfulness allow us to clear away our past experiences, trauma, unhelpful limiting beliefs and stress so our mind can navigate with ease and trust intuition and true desires, making life a much more pleasant experience. Meditation helps get us out of our primitive "fight or flight" and "black or white" survival brain and into our higher creative "gray" brain functions, more closely mirroring our true selves... a powerful, limitless, joyful and healing being.

As noted before, long-term "fight or flight" stress damages the body. Physiological changes include increased blood pressure and heart rate, wearing down the cardiovascular system, greater stress hormone release which impairs hormonal balance and fertility, and a weakened immune system which increases the likelihood of infections and autoimmune diseases. Continued long-term stress can also compromise repair functions, balance, and vitality, aging us quicker, sucking away the energy we need for joy and creativity, and making chronic diseases more likely.

Meditation and mindfulness allow us to shift our perceptions to more calm, flexibility, peace, and awareness. When we are focused on true experience, and not past interpretations and future possibilities, we can make more effective decisions using less energy. Less painful or strenuous decisions mean that we are less likely to trigger the "fight or flight" cascade, thereby allowing the healing parasympathetic nervous system activities to occur without interruption.

With practice, meditation and mindfulness allow a deep processing and recycling of limiting beliefs, experiences, and neuroplasticity (ways of thinking and processing of information). This recycling allows your brain to function from a place of curiosity, from a place of love and goodness, from a place of compassion, and from a place of truth and intelligence. Meditation allows you to continually rediscover who you are, the person who was born beautiful and perfect.

By accepting and loving yourself and showing compassion to yourself, you can then show the same love and compassion to others, creating a microenvironment of healing and love that will spread to the macro environment if enough people engage in the activity.

As meditation allows you to release the karma of your past, the choices you base your actions on, you are better able to create a future independent of your past and you can experience a freedom never previously experienced… one a bit more like bliss.

Meditation is the perfect way to enrich your life; you experience wholeness which soothes your very being, allowing you to bring this state of calm into your life every day.

Like exercise, there are many different types of meditation. Some types of meditation and mindfulness may work better for different purposes. Later I will describe all of them in greater detail. Until then, feel free to jump ahead and use Chapter 24 as a reference for any of the meditative practices I discuss throughout the book!

During the detoxification phase, I encourage Mindfulness Based Stress Reduction (MBSR) and forgiveness meditations. These meditations work both to protect you from the stress of irrational fears and to detox out anger, hostility, and resentment. These unwanted emotional qualities keep the brain functioning at the primitive level, preventing higher brain functions and the creation of a healing internal environment.

During the nourishing phase, I recommend loving kindness meditation and Kundalini mantra meditations.

During the activate phase I love Primordial Sound Meditation (PSM) or Transcendental Meditation methods, which allow you to raise your consciousness to a higher level.

As you meditate….

Meditation in general helps with mindfulness by improving your brain's ability to disregard frivolous information. By frivolous information I mean unhelpful thoughts and emotions. Meditation is a workout tool for your brain. It helps you understand that just because these thoughts come from inside your head, they are not you! Furthermore, these thoughts do not represent reality or know anything about absolute truths. Learning how to be mindful will help you assess situations at hand and put them into perspective without un-useful emotion or unproductive thoughts or fears.

Meditation helps decrease your body's reaction to stress. Those who practice it regularly begin to output less stress hormones when encountering perceived stressful events. This means the next time you are taking an exam, are working on an important project, or are dealing with a difficult individual, your body will not physically react, preserving otherwise compromised healthy functions.

Meditation and the practice of being mindful allow you to live free from past and present brain wiring (based on experience or emotion). It gives you the opportunity to live with full attention and intention. You can finally be free to choose your actions and reactions, giving you the control to act per your true values and goals. This is super useful when you must speak or work with someone you are normally emotionally charged toward. Your mindful meditation practice will allow you to engage in difficult situations with much more control, avoiding the use of regrettable actions or words.

For myself, I can thank my mindfulness practice for allowing me to handle difficult conversations with my loved ones more elegantly, without bringing up unhealthy past emotions and avoiding unproductive correspondence. I also find working with difficult clients or patients is easier as I can work harder to be fully present, compassionate and humble for them as they share their concerns, not assuming I know the reasoning behind their symptoms, behavior, or illness. This presence has allowed me to do much better work, helping me stay open and supportive, so that I can provide the best environment for the person I am helping to heal.

Meditation and mindfulness help you act more intentionally, and with purpose. This allows you to learn to engage in other life activities more productively. Activities such as eating, driving, exercising, bathing, and speaking are done with more care and effectiveness. You begin to eat healthier as you begin to identify when you are *really* hungry and when you are misreading other emotions, such as being tired, irritable, sad, or anxious, for needing food. Being mindful around food can help prevent overeating and feelings of guilt and judgments in association with the act. (To learn more about this, see my post on "Eating with your mind" in the blog section of ABeautifulRx.com.)

You also begin to move better as you start to pay attention to how you move, how intensely you move, and the skill you use in performing movements. You can prevent accidents, burn more calories, and shape your body better while you're at it.

The practice of meditation, and the resulting mindfulness we adopt, can help us live life with an attitude of kindness and flexibility of perception. We consequentially realize that there is no "right way of thinking." We must be able to adapt and change our way of thinking as we move through life.

In fact, it's better *not* to have a strategy of thinking, but instead to act authentically as you live your life.

Understanding this concept of "baby/gummy brain" will allow you to connect with a wider variety of people. This is the resilient brain that can be achieved because of practicing meditation. Thinking like a baby will allow you to genuinely give others the benefit of the doubt, put yourself in their shoes, and accept others despite differences in perspectives. Baby/gummy brain will, ultimately, increase your creativity in every situation. This newfound creativity will allow you to be less judgmental and less stressed in the presence of those who challenge your old way of thinking, and help you discover solutions where you previously could not see them.

Finally, practicing meditation and mindfulness will allow you to know yourself better. By being able to clear up your head and reach down into your core belief system, you will be able to identify your values and life objectives better.

The ability to know who you are, why you act in a certain way, and where you want to go will make life so much easier and more pleasant to navigate. You will be able to make decisions faster and get less stressed in the process. Your relationships will improve as you can explain yourself better and more confidently.

Ultimately, you will become socially and emotionally intelligent and make better decisions about how and with whom you interact. This clarity of values will help get your actions in line with your beliefs, improving your ability to act in a way that favors your health and wellbeing (my favorite part!).

Chapter 12

Anchored in Your Potential

Each of us is born with the gift of healing. We can help ourselves heal and we can help each other to heal. We just need to be made aware of this gift and learn how to use it. (Unknown Author)

Knowing your healing is essential, not only for your ability to thrive but also for your ability to uplift and serve others to your maximum capacity. We often believe sacrifice is necessary to help others when in fact self-care is more effective in the long term. Abandoning your own health and happiness will always catch up to you, resulting in irregular mood, illness and toxic drama. You are truly the only person you can effectively and predictably transform and impact.

If you miss the opportunity to create harmony in our own mind and life, you may miss the opportunity to create this for any other living person. By healing yourself, you free up extra love, creativity and energy to address the needs of others in the most empowering and healing way.

Healing must be self-initiated or it will not be sustainable. You must seek to teach by experience and tools, not by giving people remedies that they cannot apply when you are not there.

The exception to this is when we have acute diseases, infections, injuries, or advanced disease. These of course require expert delivery of whatever solution is necessary to get us out of danger.

The bottom line is this. Know you have all the qualities of your most cherished and beloved healers, teachers and leaders. You just need to remove the barriers, nourish yourself appropriately, and share your journey with those you love or seek to inspire!

Chapter 13

The Transformational Mindset

Now that you have all the background into what it takes to keep your body, mind and spirit healthy, it's time to prepare you for the Return to Beautiful Journey itself. The experience I have created is based on a philosophy of health optimization. This philosophy was made with love and a holistic spirit, infusing my cross-cultural medical and life wisdom. Health optimization has, of course, physical, emotional, mental, and spiritual aspects. I have researched this strategy over the last decade and found wisdom from my vast education.

Information and tools were sourced from institutions (Duke Integrative Medicine, Center of Mind-Body Medicine, Institute of Functional and Integrative Medicine), master teachers (Deepak Chopra, Gabrielle Bernstein, Dr. Demartini), and the schools of healing and medicine (Yoga, Meditation, Traditional Chinese Medicine, Ayurveda, Anti-aging medicine).

While working on my doctorate, I learned how to research and write on global health and environmental health issues and was able to see first-hand how effective systems of disease prevention were developed. Studying global health and the alarming rise of chronic disease linked to stress, mood disorders, chemicals, poor nutrition, and violence, I decided to dedicate much of my research and clinical work to finding strategies to stop the madness.

I wanted to focus on the healing, not on the disease. I wanted to focus on empowering the patient. I wanted it to be a system of not only disease prevention but a method that could be used to promote flourishing health. I wanted to clear up the suffering around health and open the door to a more blissful existence.

I knew that much of today's medicine was focused on managing disease and I knew that if we focused on removing barriers to a highly functioning body and nourishing a beautiful life, disease resistance would be high and healthcare more efficient.

In 2012, I began to test my strategies as I launched **The Clean and Beautiful Reset**, an ultimate health reboot program, from which the backbone of this book was created. I saw miracles occur in my patients. They were not only healthier (had on average 70% less symptoms, lost weight, had more energy, were less moody and were sleeping better), but they were more joyous and they felt by the end of their journey with me that they too now had a mission: to heal and teach their loved ones how to live a more blissful life.

My goal with **The Clean and Beautiful Reset** was to infuse spirituality and mind-body medicine into the way I cared for patients. I wanted their treatments to be as beautiful as they were... as beautiful as life could be.

"Looking at beauty in the world is the first step of purifying the mind."
— Amit Ray, *Meditation: Insights and Inspirations*

My wish was for people to embrace health maintenance as a creative tool for manifesting their most beautiful lives. Beauty is the manifestation of the soul. Those who perceive it are in line with who they are, and more importantly their body's function and appearance mimic the level of beauty they perceive. Beauty in the context of this book includes all characteristics of health, including synergy, radiance, infinite possibility, flow, positivity, love, creativity, light in the darkness, hope, faith, peace, joy and vitality.

"Youth is happy because it has the capacity to see beauty. Anyone who keeps the ability to see beauty never grows old."
— Franz Kafka

The more they can see the world through the lens of beautiful, the more aligned they will be with their purpose and mission, and the less influence the stress and challenges around them will impact their health. The goal is to make beauty an endpoint in all we do.... how we eat, sleep, exercise, talk to people, raise our children, move our bodies, and see the world.

In order to do this, we have some work to do. The first two of the three phases of the Return to Beautiful experience will help you get your body and mind out of the way of living in bliss. Phase 3 was created to move you from healthy to flourishing and to maximize your potential on both the physical and conscious planes.

The method is quite simple. It consists of shifting into and through three phases of health maintenance during your whole life. The duration of the first two phases depends on how far you have gotten from your ideal health vision.

In the clinic, I lead people through two weeks of detoxification-focused Phase 1, and then two weeks of repair- and nourishment-focused Phase 2. This gives the patient enough time to give the body a break from regular life's toxic overloads, ingrain healthier habits, and recycle the gut microbiome. The microbiome is the roughly 100 trillion microorganisms that reside in your body and have much to do with how you feel and function. Your experience the first couple of times putting yourself through the Phase 1 and 2 journey will allow you to decide how long you need to regain your energy, balanced mood, and healthy digestion before going to Phase 3. In general, Phase 1 and 2 should never be done in less than 21 days.

By the 3rd phase you will already feel empowered, feel more in control of your eating behaviors and "willpower," have more energy, and in general be ready to take bigger steps toward the life you have always wanted. I believe no one should make any major life decisions or take on any major challenges until in Phase 3.

Phase 3 will continue indefinitely. The more natural Phase 1 and 2 feel and the better your handle on stress management and self-care, the longer you will be able to stay in Phase 3.

This said, it's important to note that even the best of us "fall off the wagon" and need to start in Phase 1 again. A traumatic event, a period of heightened work or relationship stress, a few parties or weddings, or a long holiday can all be precursors to a series of events that leave your mind, body and spirit in jeopardy of disarray and therefore prone to premature aging, disease and life stagnation. When you start to feel, you are once again not in control of your health, choices and future, it's time to start Phase 1 again.

The point of the Return to Beautiful is to set you up for a lifetime of graceful ups and downs and to know there is a time for detoxification, nourishment, and activation of self to keep moving blissfully forward in your life. I hope this philosophy gives you comfort, knowing that all phases are necessary and can be beautiful.

Additionally, I desire to help you feel that life should not be a struggle but a dance, and that just knowing the familiar rhythms can help you understand and connect with yourself, which will help you to heal yourself and to heal others.

Most importantly I pray that you are inspired to commit to yourself, your health and your life, knowing your importance to everyone else you can impact in this love-thirsty world. Self-love and self-care are so much easier when you understand the untapped beauty you have inside of you and that the practice of returning to that core beauty daily will help you unleash your most healthy and vibrant life.

I hope that by the end of the book you believe you are a gift to us all and that we need you to use the experience created in this book to actively unleash it, fuel it and share it with us!

In reality, I want to give you all a chance to feel bliss... to feel ready to dive deeper into the meaning of life and serve to your highest potential. I do believe that after getting the body out of the way, you can focus on reaching the higher levels of awareness and consciousness where the beauty will be inevitable.

How do you know you need to Return to Beautiful?

Knowing when to start your Return to Beautiful process is easy. It's the moment you feel you have no control over your thoughts, your mood and your body. It's the moment you feel swollen, heavy, confused or like you're giving up on feeling and looking your best. It's the moment you feel you are aging and life looks a little less bright. It's the moment you start being "realistic" and less hopeful or creative with your life vision. It's the moment you are exhausted, sleeping poorly, and not excited when you wake up in the morning.

Ideally, the Return to Beautiful process will be practiced with each change of season. Since we are always changing, it's a good idea to put you through the experience just to reset your body and align yourself with the energy of the season and the person you currently are or are trying to become.

As we go through life, we change. We are never the same person. Our cells are recycled, our thoughts evolve, and our desires match our current mindset. Since we are also a product of our relationships, our education, our life events and our environment, we are constantly being challenged and nourished, metamorphosing into someone who hopefully looks like the person we always knew we were in our hearts.

It's important to get to know ourselves as we grow, making time for self-exploration, self-awareness and reflection. The Return to Beautiful experience is a perfect way to get to know yourself, making time for cleaning up, nourishment, and waking up the body in several ways, allowing you to see what serves you, or what doesn't serve you, during this chapter of your life.

For women wishing to begin Return to Beautiful, I suggest you start preparing for the experience the week after your period and start the detoxification phase mid cycle.

Chapter 14

Success in Your
Return to Beautiful Experience

Success is definitely relative, but I promise one thing; the more of the tips you adapt from the journey I have created for you, the more you will learn about yourself and the more you will transform. If you are wishing for a change, then you will have one. Watch yourself as you lead yourself through this cleansing and nourishing process. Notice each week what experiences give you the most joy, energy, and feelings of empowerment and love. The more positive energy you receive from the method, the more valuable the method is for you.

The journey was created to allow you to experience different tools of health activation. Some will respond to different tools and methods better than others. It's important to understand that some may be more powerful for you at this moment of your life. I suggest that you journal the way you feel throughout your journey as you experiment with each of these tools and lifestyle modifications. Keep a journal by your bed at night and ask yourself the following questions:

- Did you sleep well last night?

- Did you have any time to relax?

- Did you get any exercise in?

- Did you get to stretch?

- Did you get healthy communication in?

- How did you alleviate stress?

- What was your overall impression of today?

- What did you do well (that made you proud or happy)?

- What is one thing you would like to improve on?

Each day...

Write down which of these emotions best describe your day.

Energetic	Balanced	Relaxed
Optimistic	Compassionate	Sad
Loving	Creative	Frustrated
Playful	Aware	Upset
Happy	Grateful	Worried
Forgiving	Honest	Fearful
Expressive	Joyful	Stressed
Authentic	Self-accepting	Anxious
Appreciative	Solution Oriented	Depressed

How do you think your diet affected your overall mood? What else affected your disposition?

Chapter 15

Find Your Purpose and Serve the World

What is the key to flourishing health and bliss? Build a life you are truly grateful for.

We've already discussed the benefits of gratitude. Giving daily thanks for your life, the people and experiences that contribute to it, and the divine creator of it can be one of the most powerful tools to maintain health.

This said, only authentic gratitude will work. You must truly be grateful, not simply giving gratitude to reap the benefits. To do this you must do the work to find out who you truly are, what your passions are, and what your purpose is.

Once you have aligned your life with these self-discoveries you will have much to be authentically grateful for, despite the challenges and inevitable hardships.

For this reason, taking time to explore these core questions can be one of the most essential first steps for a flourishing life. One of the books that helped me realize this was Dr. Demartini's book *Inspired Destiny*. He explores values and purpose by asking these simple questions.

1. What do you fill your space with? Look at your professional and personal space and notice what you fill it with. Books, magazine, figures, pictures? What are these items about? Sports, art, travel, medicine, history, yoga, animals?

Describe the three themes that you see filling up your space in a single word.

A._____

B._____

C._____

2. How do you spend your time? No matter how busy we think we are, how we spend our time says something about who we are and what is important to us. There is always a choice and for this reason writing down how many hours a day we spend in each waking activity can help clarify for us how we choose to spend our time.

   A. I spend the most time …

   (at work, with my kids, taking care of my home, traveling, etc.)

   _____

   B. I spend the second most time …

   (reading, studying, cooking, etc.)

   _____

   C. I spend the third most time …

   (exercising, connecting with friends, etc.)

   _____

3. What energizes you the most? No matter how tired you are, you always have energy for these things.

   A._____

   B._____

   C._____

4. How do you spend most of your money? You will always spend money on that which is the most important to you.

A._____

B._____

C._____

5. What are you the most organized in? Where do you have the highest degree of order in your life? Name the three things you always seem to have in order even if other areas seem quite out of sorts. (Home, workouts, eating, finances, clothing, social events...?)

A._____

B._____

C._____

6. Where are you the most reliable, disciplined and focused? (Business, working out, family, social media, appearance, eating...?)

A._____

B._____

C._____

7. What do you inwardly think about the most? Thoughts about what you want in life can be very telling about who you are. Write down what your mind naturally loves to think about... *not what you* "should do" or "have to do" but the things you dream about! Is it a family lifestyle, riches, traveling, inspiring others, creating something...?

A._____

B._____

C._____

8. What do you always desire to talk about at parties? What you choose to speak about at parties is very indicative of your passions, as you are spending your free quality time desiring to communicate about what you love. What conversations immediately take you from introvert mode to extrovert? Is it injustice, poetry, movies, relationships, health, politics, business, travel...? Name the top three things.

A._____

B._____

C._____

9. What inspires you the most? Name certain things, experiences, people that have repeatedly made the biggest impact on you. Is it philanthropy in a certain area? Is it children's achievements? Sports? Or something else?

A._____

B._____

C._____

10. What do you easily manifest in your life? Which type of long-term goals has come true for you? Name the three most persistent goals that you have worked on and in which have started to see the fruits of your labor. (Family, career, home, athletic goal, travel, love, friendships, community, etc.?)

A._____

B._____

C._____

11. What are you constantly researching, reading about, and looking up online?

A._____

B._____

C._____

12. By looking at how you answer these questions, you can identify your values. Are these values truly aligned with your authentic self? Are you living per your own values or someone else's/society's values?

Incongruence can mean illness, unhappiness and pain for you and those around you. It can also mean you are living way below your potential.

For more a more thorough examination, I encourage you to check out Dr. Demartini's values workshop, which is offered all over the world! *Or,* you can take his online quiz, which gives more detail about the inquisitive questions that uncover your values (https://drdemartini.com/account/value-determination). If you do this, please mention this *Return to Beautiful book* as your referral source!

Once you start and focus on living a virtuous life in alignment with your gifts, passions and purpose, you will be authentically grateful and live in more flow and bliss. Again, authentic gratitude has been shown to improve wellbeing and clinical outcomes in those with heart failure, showing the connection between this feeling of deep-rooted love and your health.

Are you ready to begin? Turn the page to see the blueprint for your *Return to Beautiful* journey!

Part Two

The Journey Begins

Don't

Do It, Say It, *or* Think It

Unless It's

Healing,
Loving,
or Beautiful

Chapter 16

Phase 0: Get Ready to Return to Beautiful

So let's get into it! Let's prep you for your experience! Getting ready is very important to the success of your body and life reset… the return to your most beautiful state of being. This experience is meant to encourage extreme self-care. The more of the recommendations you adopt, the more transformational the experience will be!

This said, you may not be able to experiment with all lifestyle recommendations your first go-around. But whatever you don't get to this time, you can try in the future. Since the "Return to Beautiful" experience is meant to be repeated on an as-needed basis throughout life, you will have opportunities to build your healing, flourishing and bliss-promoting tool kit.

Below are the steps you need to take to get ready for the first phase of your journey.

Phase 0 is about getting ready. Here are my suggestions:
1. Stop eating the following foods immediately:
    a. Genetically modified foods (GMOs, all foods not labeled non-GMO)
    b. Pesticide-ridden foods (those foods non-organic and listed with warning on the EWG.org website)
    c. Gluten-containing foods (breads, pasta, cereal, cakes)
    d. Corn, sugar or sugar alternatives, dessert foods
    e. Peanuts, tuna, swordfish, soy
    f. Canned, packaged and prepared foods

g. Any foods you have tested sensitive to or that triggers allergies

- Note on food allergies: Food allergies are those foods which your body is especially reactive to, causing harmful inflammation, disturbing your metabolism, and impairing your ability to absorb nutrients from other foods you eat.

    You are susceptible to forming food allergies when you have an inflamed gut to begin with (because of chemicals and poor food choices), and they are usually foods you eat a lot of during this period of stress and unhealthy eating/living. If you have been struggling with poor digestion, suffer from autoimmune diseases, are dealing with hormonal irregularities, have a hard time losing weight, or have other unexplained symptoms, testing yourself for food allergies can help create a more effective detoxification strategy.

    In my office, I use the ALCAT test by Cell Science and incorporate the results into my personalized nutrition, detoxification, and weight loss plans.

- Other important tests your Functional Medicine practitioner may want to order are a *micronutrient* panel or genetic mutation in those genes responsible for assuring proper detoxification.

    A micronutrient deficiency can make it difficult for you to feel energized or well during your attempt to restore your health. If you have symptoms such as fatigue, resistant weight loss, bruising, bone brittleness, nervous system deficits, or hair, nail, or skin findings, finding out which vitamins or minerals you are deficient in can help your doctor find a solution quicker.

- If you have suffered from mood disorders, high blood homocysteine levels, folate deficiency, had a miscarriage, suffer from longstanding gastrointestinal complaints, or have other previously unexplained or vague symptoms, getting tested for genetic polymorphisms (mutant variants) may be helpful.

  In my clinic, I test for Methylenetetrahydrofolate Reductase (MTHFR), an important enzyme necessary for methylation, DNA repair, and gene modulation. MTHFR is essential for folate and folic acid conversion to active 5-methyltetrahydrofolate (5-MTHF), and the ability to produce neurotransmitters such as serotonin, dopamine and catecholamines (i.e. epinephrine).

  Ultimately, lack of MTHFR puts you at risk for a host of health conditions, including heart disease, fertility issues, Alzheimer's and cancer. Those on medications such as antacids, metformin, or high blood pressure medications, who are also positive for MTHFR mutation, could be at increased risk of complications and should therefore discuss this with physician and consider being tested as well.

- Catechol-O-methyltransferase (COMT) is another important enzyme that is responsible for degradation of catecholamines, putting patients at risk for epinephrine buildup and symptoms such as aggression, anger and anxiety. COMT gene mutations are also being explored for associated with impulsiveness, poor decision-making, ADHD and autism. COMT suppression can also occur with environmental attributes such as exposure to endocrine disruptors, such as BPAs or mercury toxicity.

To rule out any genetic mutations, seek out your Functional Medicine expert and get more personalized guidance, as these mutations can be easily managed with therapeutic supplementation and diet modification. Please feel free to contact me at Jelena@mybeautifulgenetics.com for more information on testing or referrals. *The Institute of Functional Medicine* also has a list of certified practitioners in your area who are well versed in specialized testing and integrative management of conditions and disease prevention.

2. Focus on whole foods, a rainbow of colors. Avoid most processed carbohydrates. See the Shopping List (in Chapter 31 Section A). It is important to buy the right "clean" organic fats, proteins, and seeds to support your reset. Eating high quality foods is especially important during this experience. Remember, the more you do, the more transformative this health and life reset will be.

3. Prepare for lifestyle homework: As mentioned, each week you will get some lifestyle homework asking you to experience a different stress-relieving or health-enhancing activity. I encourage you to try them out and see which ones can shift your perspective and help you (a) feel more in tune with your true self, (b) relax and enjoy life more, (c) achieve mental clarity and decision making power, (d) have more energy, and (f) enhance creativity and feelings of excitement.

4. Starting today, I advise you to tell everyone who can impact the success of your journey that you are preparing to reset your health and your life.

- Do not forget family, friends and other important figures in your life, such as your boss or coworkers. These people can serve to offer you both support and accountability, increasing your success during this experience.

5. Use the Journal Page in Chapter 31 Section B as a guide to note important shifts in your energy, mood, hunger and emotions during your journey.

6. I also strongly recommend using the *Wellness Activity Checklist* (Chapter 31 Section D) to keep track of your wellness activities. You can also download it and other helpful documents from ABeautifulRx.com. You will find it in the *Return to Beautiful* tab. I encourage you to take wellness seriously and make sure to use the assigned lifestyle activities daily to maximize the results of this reset.

7. Start to pay attention, breathe, and look at things with curiosity and a "beginner's" mind. Start to question if what you are doing, eating, or planning falls in line with your ideal health/life/beauty vision. Decisions will get easier the more you check in and question your actions. During each phase of this journey to your best self and life, I will give you some helpful tips on how to keep your environment from challenging your health, wellness, and happiness. It is not fair that you are working hard to fuel and nurture your mind and body, while environmental elements are simultaneously polluting them.

8. The day before your Phase 1 start date, partake in an optional liquid fast.

- When you wake up, drink a cup of warm filtered water with fresh lemon squeezed into it.
- Next sip on a cup of fresh grapefruit juice with a spoonful of MCT (medium chain triglycerides) oil (or organic castor oil) between 9 and 10 am. Please check with your physician if you are on any prescription medications that could possibly interact with grapefruit juice. If so, a green juice (3 green veggies to 1 green apple or pear) would be a good alternative.
- After this, sip on a variety of organic teas and infusions throughout the day. You can use lemon and ginger to spice your green tea, mint tea, ginger tea, chamomile tea or other favorite herbal tea.
- For lunch, have 2 cups of spiced broth (homemade is best but otherwise organic premade is okay). Spiced broth is simply broth made with a variety of spices, garlic and onion (if not sensitive) and olive oil.

> **Teas and Coffees**
>
> Tea and coffee are some of the most pesticide ridden commercially grown plants on the planet. This reason for this is that they are high commodity and can be sold for a high price around the globe. Those drinking coffee and tea mindlessly (without considering if organic and not considering the quantity ingested) can suffer tremendously from both digestive and liver function. In addition, those who have issues detoxifying coffee (slow metabolizers) suffer from over activation of the adrenals and over acidification and oxidation (leaching nutrients as it remains in the system over an extended period of time).

- As an early evening snack have vegetable-dominant green juice. Vegetable dominant means 3 vegetables for 1 green apple, 1 green pear or 1 kiwi.
- For dinner, have another 2 cups of broth.
- Have a cup of herbal tea before you go to bed.

9. Order any supplements recommended in the Supplement List chapter. None are necessary but all are highly recommended, as they make sure your liver is well supported and that you feel your best during your detoxification. I work with only the cleanest supplements that have universal health benefits. See my supplement list for an explanation of when and how they should be used. All my readers can use a special code for discounts off supplements. The code is RTB15 and is for a 15% discount.

Now that you know what you are in for... let's start this!

Chapter 17

Phase 1: Detox Out Barriers to Health

Week 1 - Diet

This week we are focusing on removing all inflammatory foods.

- As recommended in Phase 0, remove foods such as gluten, soy, dairy, corn, wheat, packaged/premade foods, canned foods, sugars and sugar alternatives, peanuts, GMO and non-organic foods, and tuna and other high mercury fish. These foods are never helpful, but during this experience it's essential we remove them. The body cannot fully recover and heal from "regular living" without the full removal of these foods. They promote inflammation in the digestive tract and, in general, cause inflammation throughout the body, triggering stress, making nutrient absorption difficult. These foods also are more likely to harbor chemicals or feed microorganisms, such as yeast and gas-producing bacteria, making optimal function difficult.

- Bake 2 sweet potatoes and cook 3 cups of quinoa and refrigerate ahead of time if you want to have these in your first weeks of the experience.

- Pea protein shakes for the detox as well as the detox support supplements can be bought on my website's on-line store (ABeautifulRx.com/shop) and are known as the Paleo Cleanse 14-day kit. Other supplements can also be purchased as described in the program.

Week 1 and 2: Holistic Detox

General Guidelines: *No Soy, Corn, Wheat, Gluten, Sugar or Alternative, Dairy, Coffee, packaged or store-bought food, high-mercury fish (tuna and swordfish), farmed fish, conventional produce and animal products, peanuts, or alcohol.*

Focus On: *Whole foods, Supplements, Spices, Non-GMO, and Organic foods.*

For those trying to lose weight, look at the green highlighted recommended supplements.

Overview
- Wellness
- Sweat in the AM
- Jump in a pool of water
- Move before and after each meal
- Stop negative thoughts
- Don't gossip or complain
- Remove yourself from negative people and environments
- Forgiveness Meditation
- Shaking and Dancing Meditation
- Conversation about your past
- Ego Eradicator

The Plan - Week 1

Pre-Breakfast Upon Waking	• Juice of 1 Organic Lemon in a large 12-ounce glass of filtered water + ½ tsp. Vitamin C Bio Fizz (at least 500mg) • Take These Supplements: Omega 3 supplements + PGX (2 capsules) + Vitamin D (if tested and deficient)
AM Activity Sweat	Shaking and Dancing Meditation (Chapter 24)/Sauna/Physical activity 20-30 min minimum **NOTE:** *Only add physical activity if you feel it will not compromise your diet. Most first-timers may want to focus the first few days of this detox phase on adapting to diet and lifestyle.*
Breakfast Before 9 AM	• Paleo Cleanse Protein Shake (Protein of non-GMO yellow pea protein) with ice + water or non-dairy milk + spinach + berries + dash of cinnamon, turmeric, ginger and cayenne pepper optional. **NOTE:** *Cayenne pepper not indicated for those with heartburn, irritable bowel, ulcers or other severe digestive issues. Please see your doctor for questions.* • Detox Supplement Pack – amino acids and digestive enzymes
Between Breakfast and Lunch	• Organic Green Tea – Sip a cup or two between meals • 3 glasses of filtered water. May take PGX fiber (2 capsules, buy at Whole Foods or online for extra bowel support or to help control hunger or sugar addictions). • 15-minute Vitamin D break. Go outside and seek the sun. The best times are 10 AM to 3 PM.
Lunch before 3: 10 Soft Belly Breaths	• Organic, non-GMO plant or animal proteins, wild fish + rainbow of veggies • If needed, ½ sweet potato or quinoa • Curcumin – 800 mg
Between Lunch and Dinner	• Organic herbal tea (ginger or mint best) • 3 glasses of filtered water • PGX fiber (2 capsules)
PM Activity	Walk 20 min. Ideal time for *Ego Eradicator/Forgiveness Meditation (Chapter 24)*

The Plan - Week 1 *cont.*

Dinner **Before 8 PM**	• Shake with cinnamon and kale • Detox Supplement Pack • Colon Rx • Magnesium Citrate powder (300 mg or 1 spoon in a glass of water)
Before Sleep	• **No electronics after dinner. Relaxing music and inspirational reading.** • Sleep before 10 PM. Body best detoxifies and rejuvenates between 10 PM and 2 AM.

Lifestyle Details – Week 1

MOVEMENT: Think about sweating. Many chemicals are easily removed through the skin via sweating!

Using a sauna, if not ready to exercise	Especially if you are a smoker, adding in 1-3 sessions of sauna this week can accelerate the detoxifying process. Make sure you start out with only a few minutes. If you are under the care of a healthcare provider, seek their permission first. Infrared saunas are the best type as they heat from the inside out and help purge everything out through the skin. **NOTE** *Try taking a refreshing shower right after your sauna experience and feel the energy and lightness you gain.*
Spinning, Running, Bikram yoga	• At the very least walk fast for 30 minutes minimum first thing in the morning are great ways to break a sweat and activate the body. • Try to get up and move 10 minutes before and after each meal. • Try not to eat at your desk. • Get up to stretch, and make your lunch spot a destination you must get up and move to reach. Moving after your meals can help aid digestion and promote better bowel motility. • Make it a habit to move after each meal and improve your overall wellbeing, nutrient absorption and detoxification!
Breakfast Before 9 AM	• Paleo Cleanse Protein Shake (Protein of non-GMO yellow pea protein) with ice + water or non-dairy milk + spinach + berries + dash of cinnamon, turmeric, ginger and cayenne pepper optional. **NOTE:** *Cayenne pepper not indicated for those with heartburn, irritable bowel, ulcers or other severe digestive issues. Please see your doctor for questions.* • Detox Supplement Pack – amino acids and digestive enzymes

Emotional/Mental Fitness – Week 1

If possible, once this week try this to help break up neuroplasticity. Neuroplasticity is when your mind gets fixated on one type of thought process or belief that keeps you stuck on a habit, a way of thinking or living that holds you back from making positive changes in your life.

Jump in a pool of water, the ocean, or another body of water
• Submerge yourself underwater, and as you rise above the surface notice how you feel. How did the rest of your day go? What else did you notice? Cool or cold water seems to have an extra advantage in shifting perspectives, making more room for creativity. **NOTE** *Can't get into a pool? Take a bath and try floating and submerging your head a few times. It's not as effective but it can shift things for you.* • Try this out when feeling negative, stuck or unable to decide about something important to you.
Have a game plan for negative thoughts
One I use when a negative thought comes through is to say "next." Use your mantra of choice, such as "I am enough," "I am light," or "I am love." Stopping negative thoughts as they enter your mind can be quite tedious at first but you will notice the more you stop them the less frequently they will come!
Make a vow to not gossip or complain
Keep yourself accountable. Draw on the superior portion of your fist this symbol * (or another type of star), reminding you of your potential and purpose and of how complaining and gossip is not in line with your mission!
Consider removing yourself from negative environments
If there are certain people in your life who engage in these activities or are especially negative, this is an opportunity to explain to them how this can impact your health negatively. Take a good look at the people in your life and decide who is not serving and supporting your expansion as a person.

Emotional/Mental Fitness – Week 1 *cont.*

Forgive
• The Forgiveness Meditation (described in Chapter 24) can help you release blame and anger toward yourself or others quickly! • Use the Forgiveness Meditation twice a day for 2 minutes to heal a relationship that is weighing heavily on your heart. If you can find no other moment, try practicing it while brushing your teeth!
• **Detox out tension and emotion in your tissues**
The Shaking and Dancing Meditation (Chapter 24). I often find this type of meditation especially helpful when I am stressed out. Sometimes you just need to shake sh** out!   *I thank my teachers at the Center of Mind-Body Medicine (https://cmbm.org/) for introducing me to this technique… I even get my kids to do the dance variety when the household environment gets especially tense.*   *Dr. James Gordon, a Harvard trained psychiatrist and founder of the Center of Mind-Body Medicine, learned this from an Eastern Medicine healer and now helps people across the world suffering from anxiety, depression, and fear with this method.*
Clear Up/Be Okay with Your Past
Life Exploration Conversation • Over the weekend, block off a good 2 hours with a good non-judgmental friend. Find someone supportive and communicate to them your past and how it has shaped and impacted you. Touch on how you have grown stronger and what you have learned through your experiences. Discuss letting go and embracing your authentic self. Tell them who you are, what is important to you, and your life objective.   *This exercise can be very detoxifying and build confidence in your journey. It is important to let your friend know you need them to listen more than anything. What is important is not any advice or opinions they may offer, but what you notice about yourself as they discuss your life. Your reaction to what is said during this conversation can help you know yourself better. Pay attention and see how you can use this to make better decisions*

Emotional/Mental Fitness – Week 1 *cont.*

- If you are open to it, consider consulting with a Hypnotist or Energy Healer.
- I have used both. For someone with deep-rooted pain from a traumatic event, a troubled childhood, or family dynamics, it may take assistance to clear these things quickly.

  Hypnotists can help pinpoint the moment when you may have begun to develop stress or certain beliefs which have been holding you back from progressing in life or healing from a physical or mental ailment.

  Energy healers similarly can find blocks which you've accumulated in your body along the chakras which could be preventing you from feeling free of pain, negativity, fear or deep-rooted beliefs which make progressing into a better life very difficult. I personally have generations of post-traumatic stress from hardships related to war, poverty, prejudice and limiting beliefs that held me back for years. In a single session with an energy healer I felt liberated from a deep heaviness I always felt inside.

  This said, not all hypnotists and energy workers are created equal. I would be very careful only to use those recommended by trusted sources. If you need me to recommend someone, I have a few trusted experts I can whole-heartedly recommend.

Get the ego out of the way

- My last recommendation is a Kundalini kriya called the Ego Eradicator.
- What is the ego? The ego is a false sense of ourselves we develop over our lifetime that is shaped by what we have come to believe to be true after years of programming by others, society, and the interpretation of life events and experiences. The ego is our self-image and is formed by judgments by others and ourselves. When our ego is in the way, we cannot see our true selves and we are limited in our possibilities and in our creativity. The way we can see beyond the lens of our ego and become aligned with our true self is through practices of mindfulness and awareness. Meditation helps us recognize our true self and recycle out karma that energizes the ego. Meditation also helps us develop the habit of recognizing thoughts, behaviors and other sensory inputs for what they simply distractions, and not in any way related to our true limitless nature.
- My last recommendation is a Kundalini kriya called the Ego Eradicator.

Emotional/Mental Fitness – Week 1 *cont.*

- Kriya means action that works to facilitate a desired outcome. In Kundalini yoga, a kriya is a series of postures, breathing, and sounds that work to help transform you physically and mentally to make your desires more likely to occur. Depending on the kriya you use, you can support various organs, neural pathways, the hormone system, the circulatory system, the spine, and other vital processes in the body to function optimally. Kriyas help tone the mind, body and spirit so that you function better as a whole.

- The Ego Eradicator kriya is a simple and effective exercise to get yourself out of the way of your healing. The exercise consists of holding the posture shown below for 3 - 5 minutes while breathing rapidly in and out of your nose. The breathing technique is called the "Breath of Fire" and it is often used in yoga classes to help detoxify the body.

  - Sit in an easy cross-legged pose on the floor. Sit on a pillow under your tailbone for support and make sure you are pulling your abdomen in as you pull up your body comfortably straight, allowing your vertebral column to stretch up from the base of your tailbone and up your back and through your neck to the top of your head. Hold out your arms at a 60-degree angle in a V formation and stick your thumbs up while bending your other fingers toward your palm.

- Begin to breathe as rapidly as you can in and out of your nose, pulsing your belly button in with each inhalation. Hold this pose for 3 - 5 minutes.

- The Ego Eradicator is best done on an empty stomach. It should be repeated daily for 20 days for best results.

- Try this with the song Gobinda by Mirabai Ceiba. You can find it on my Spotify list (Jelena Ley Petkovic) under Shaking and Dancing Meditations.

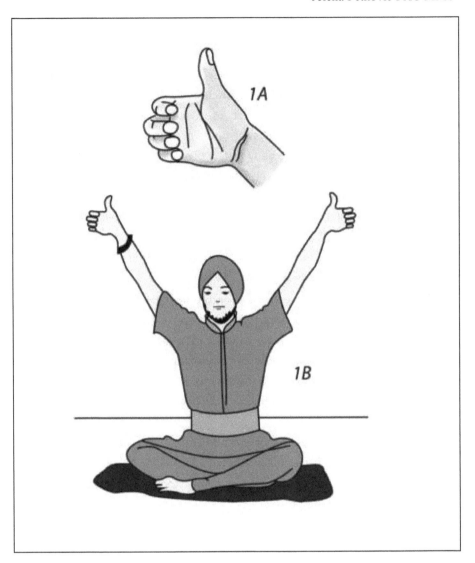

Ego Eradicator

The Plan - Week 2 Holistic Detox

Overview

- Wellness
- Start cardio
- Don't use electronics when eating or close to sleeping
- Buy a water filter
- Switch to safer cosmetics, creams, shampoos and make-up
- Stop using perfumes
- Avoid BPA: Plastics, cookware and receipts
- Prepare broths and breakfast for Phase 2

Lifestyle Details – Week 2

Diet	• Continue the diet prescribed in week 1. For any questions, you have up to this point, please feel free to contact me on ABeautifulRx.com/contact.
	• By this week you should be deep in the groove of your Return to Beautiful experience. If you haven't already, add in some supplements to support your detoxification efforts. Add Omega 3 fatty acids, curcumin, PGX fiber, and Ayurvedic herbs for colon health (Colon Rx on ABeautifulRx.com). Add some non-GMO yellow pea protein shakes (see Paleo Cleanse Shakes on ABeautifulRx.com), and some liver support (see Hepatatone or the Paleo Cleanse Packets in the Paleo Cleanse Detox Kit). These supplements help decrease inflammation, support the immune system and liver, and support vitality.
	• If you wish to speed your metabolism, use the tips below. Metabolism Boosting Tips:
	    ○ Drink warm liquid throughout the day. Add lemon and ginger to stimulate digestion and cleansing.
	    ○ Walk 20 minutes after each meal.

Lifestyle Details – Week 2 *cont.*

Diet	o Make lunch your heaviest meal. Have a small dinner. o Try not to snack, especially if one of your original complaints is low energy. This helps your body to detox. If you must snack, stick with a piece of low glycemic fruit (organic green apples or berries are best) and tea *or* a cup of broth. o Keeping hydrated will help with food withdrawals and stimulate detoxification and metabolism. o Your metabolism is at its highest between 10 AM and 3 PM, so eat lunch before 3 PM. o Eat dinner before 8 PM and be asleep by 10 PM. Sleeping between 10 PM and 2 AM is essential for fat loss and detoxification. o If you ate a large dinner, skip breakfast the next day. o If you are going out over the weekend, have an approved protein shake or a soup with lean protein for lunch, and have a dinner salad with light fish/protein and vegetables (no sauce or butter).
Movement	• Start cardio-sweat exercises if you haven't already. o The best exercises for this are those that promote sweating, such as cycling, spinning, swimming, and Bikram yoga. o During the detoxification, I recommend daily sweating. At minimum try to walk/run for a minimum of 30 minutes, first thing in the morning, three times per week. Then add in the other activities as you see possible. o The Shaking and Dancing Meditation can count as a sweating activity for those stressed for time. You should be able to squeeze that into less than 25 minutes. o Remember, don't start the exercising until you've adapted to the new diet and eating schedule, but be mindful that the more you can change your regular routine and add in these lifestyle medicine tips, the more transformational the experience will be.

Lifestyle Details – Week 2 *cont.*

Environment	• We have touched upon the importance of eating organic, non-GMO foods previously in the book. We also discussed how to avoid chemicals in the environment to the best of your ability. If you haven't already, it's time to do even more to limit toxicity in your environment. • One toxicity is being around electronics too much and too often. They ramp up our minds, making it difficult to relax our minds and effectively rejuvenate. Avoid TV and electronics while eating and after 6 PM. Eating and looking at electronics have been correlated with overeating, and eating too quickly makes both digestion and weight management difficult. Additionally, TVs and computers should never be placed in your bedroom. The bedroom should be used strictly for relaxing, sleeping and lovemaking. Electronics get in the way of all three of these vital activities. ☹ • If you don't have one already, buy a filter for your faucet. Simply drinking enough clean water can transform your health. Water can also be one of our biggest sources of toxicity, containing harmful minerals, chemicals and waste byproducts. Make sure you are drinking from non-BPA containers, especially when drinking hot liquids. My favorite filter is the Kangen water system. The Kangen system cleans the water without stripping the helpful components, can be calibrated for ideal pH, and is infused with antioxidants shown to be healing for a variety of illnesses. • Again, it's very important that anything you put on your skin, or use anywhere on your body, is as clean as possible, especially for your day to day use. Buy deodorant, face wash, shampoo, and creams that are "clean." • Perfumes are also an unfortunate cause of toxicity, containing endocrine disruptors which throw off your natural hormonal rhythms. My advice is to stick to trusted essential oil brands. I have found some dream scents, which I can use to smell lovely I

Lifestyle Details – Week 2 *cont.*

Environment	without any worry of harm to myself or others who are exposed. The Return to Beautiful experience is a perfect time to go the extra mile to avoid chemicals which could be harmful for your health! I know it may seem like a pain, but at least try it for the detox and repair portion of the experience. Stay away from artificial fragrances and personal care products! Reconsider buying conventional make-up and get familiar with brands using more natural and organic ingredients. Need help finding cleaner products? The Environmental Working Group at EWG.org and www.ewg.org/Skindeep provides a list of safer cosmetics. • If you are not already, it is now time to get BPA out of your life! Avoiding BPA means (a) looking for plastics marked non-BPA, (b) not hoarding or handling paper receipts, (c) avoiding recycled pizza boxes or toilet paper, and (d) eliminating canned goods, including sparkling and tonic water.

You coming to the end of Phase 1 and that means it's time to prep for Phase 2!

Sunday prior to the start of Phase 2:

- Browse the Supplement List and Shopping List (Chapter 31) and make sure you have all you need to get started!
- Make Chicken/Veggie Bone Broth (the recipe is in Chapter 28).
- Make 2 Cups of Steel Cut Gluten Free Oatmeal the Sunday before your Monday start.

Chapter 18

Phase 2: Nourish and Restore

Congratulations! *You* have successfully completed the detox portion of the Return to Beautiful experience.

You should feel more in control of your health, with fewer cravings for sugar and processed carbs, and in general less hungry with the nutritious food you have been incorporating into your daily diet. You also should notice a subtle new glow in your complexion, feel less inflamed, have more energy, be in a better mood, and be sleeping better. The initial anxiety surrounding your new lifestyle habits should be gone and you should be excited about continuing your health journey.

If you are not experiencing these benefits or are feeling worse, please contact your own healthcare provider. If you are in Miami, please make an appointment to see me for a more thorough examination.

The next phase is to focus on improving your gut/digestive health, increase your natural metabolism, and provide extra nourishment and love to your mind, body and spirit.

Overview - Week 3

- Wellness
- Add fermented foods
- Make sure you are getting enough good fats and spices (garlic, onion, MCT oil)
- Start probiotics
- Focus on *love* and all that nourishes it

Lifestyle Details – Week 3

Wellness	<ul><li>Gratitude Exercise</li><li>Self-Massage</li><li>Loving Kindness Meditation</li><li>Yoga</li><li>Grounding</li><li>Kundalini Mantra</li><li>Sleep Hygiene Checklist</li><li>Happiness 40 List</li><li>*Hug* every day</li><li>Contact with nature: Mindful walk, and Grounding</li></ul>
Diet	<ul><li>Focus on adding fermented foods, good fats, and spices</li><li>Switch from lemon water every morning to a shot of apple cider vinegar</li><li>Start pro/ prebiotics and fermented food before lunch every day</li><li>Use digestive enzymes if indigestion and gases are still occurring</li><li>Try to cut down on carbohydrates. Limit your beans, sweet potatoes, or quinoa serving to the days you do more cardiovascular exercise and feel a bit of anxiety creeping in.</li><li>Get garlic or onion in every lunch meal</li><li>Try to get steamed broccoli or cabbage into your diet every day (unless you are allergic!)</li><li>Alternate breakfast choices between a) gluten free oats, chia seed and flaxseed pudding, b) eggs and veggies, and c) yellow pea protein shake</li><li>Use coconut oil in the preparation of your breakfast, adding medium chain triglycerides (MCT coconut) into your shake with the addition of spices such as cayenne pepper, ginger and turmeric</li><li>MCT oil is food for the liver and brain, calming the nervous system and promoting vitality</li><li>The spices mentioned are anti-inflammatory, promote a healthy immune system, and aid metabolism. Make sure your sources are clean and organic, as spices can be a major source of impurities such as chemicals and heavy metals.</li></ul>

The Plan - Week 3

Pre-Breakfast Upon Waking	• Gratitude Exercise • Self-Massage Time Slot • 1 Tablespoon of apple cider vinegar + 12-ounce glass of filtered water + ½ tsp Vitamin C Bio Fizz. • Take These Supplements: Omega 3 (2), Vitamin D (3 drops)
AM Activity	Loving Kindness Meditation (Chapter 24) Move 60 min: *yoga*
Breakfast Before 9 AM	• Shake with ice + water or non-dairy milk + spinach + berries • *or* 3 egg whites + 1 egg with 3 different color veggies • *or* 3 Tablespoons GF Oats + 1 teaspoon chia seeds +1 teaspoon flax seeds + almond / coconut milk + cinnamon • PGX-2
Between Breakfast and Lunch	• Organic green tea • 3 glasses of filtered water. One glass with 1 spoonful GI Revive. • Supplements: Probiophage (or another probiotic supplement) • 15-minute Vitamin D break. Go outside and seek the sun. The best time is from 10 AM to 3 PM.
Lunch before 3: 10 soft belly breaths	• 1 spoonful kimchi and water • Organic, non-GMO plant, wild fish + rainbow of veggies • If needed, ½ sweet potato or quinoa • Curcumin – 800 mg
Between Lunch and Dinner	• Organic herbal tea (ginger or mint best) • 3 glasses of filtered water • PGX - 2
PM Activity	Walk 20 min. Mindful Nature Walk /Kundalini Mantra /Grounding activity
Dinner Before 8 PM	• Bone broth soup or blended vegetable soup. Add spices. **NOTE:** *You can eat the vegetables but do not eat the meat portion for dinner.* • 15 ounces of filtered water with 2 spoons tart cherry juice • Herbal tea

The Plan - Week 3 *cont.*

Dinner Before 8 PM	• Colon Rx-1 • Magnesium chelate or Epsom salt bath
Before Sleep	• **No electronics after dinner.** • **Relaxing music and inspirational reading.** • Self-Massage Time Slot • Gratitude PM • Sleep before 10 PM. Body best detoxifies and rejuvenates between 10 PM and 2 AM.

Lifestyle Details - Week 3

Week 3 should be about stretching, self-care practices, resting, and creating more space and calm in your life.

Focus more on *sleep hygiene.* Some recommendations by the Institute of Functional Medicine for better sleep include:
• Avoid alcohol 3 hours before sleep • Avoid caffeine after 12 noon • Avoid decongestants and cold medicine at night • Avoid exercise after 6 PM • Avoid the news or other media during dinner • Avoid naps after Noon • Avoid naps longer than 45 minutes • Avoid heavy, spicy meals at dinner • Avoid eating after dinner • Avoid drinking more than 4 - 8 ounces before sleep • Take a hot salt/aromatherapy bath before sleep. A warm shower can help too. • Adding lavender oil and Epsom salts to your bath will promote relaxation, and decrease cortisol stress hormone before sleep • Listen to relaxing music and/or read inspirational but calming reading material before sleep

Lifestyle Details - Week 3 *cont.*

For those requesting a musical sleep remedy, I usually give my patients a sleep time prayer/song to help them transition into sleep. The song I use is a peace/protection prayer Kirtan Sohila - Musical Version by Snatam Kaur. You can find it on You Tube and Spotify. Check it out and see if it resonates!

- When attempting to sleep, don't stay in bed more than 30 minutes attempting to do so. It is better to get out and return to try again.
- Make sure windows are covered well and early light cannot creep into your room and interrupt your sleep
- Close windows if noise is likely to wake you up early
- Sleep in a cool environment
- Use hypo-allergenic pillows
- Avoid waterbeds and the use of electric fields near bed
- For those who sleep on their side, consider using a side pillow, hugging a pillow, and putting it between your knees for better spinal alignment
- Sleep on the best linens that you can afford

NOTE: *For those struggling to fall asleep consider taking the following supplements:*

- o **Melatonin:** 1 - 5 mg to fall asleep or 5 - 20 mg time released to stay asleep
- o **5HTP:** 50 - 300 mg 1 hour before bedtime
- o **Taurine:** 500 - 2000 mg 1 hour before bedtime
- o **Magnesium/Calcium:** 250 - 500 mg of magnesium citrate or 400 - 800 mg of glycinate at bedtime
- o Herbal tea before bedtime can help support relaxation before rest. Try lemon balm or passion flower.

- Morning blue light therapy or 10,000 lix bright light exposure upon waking can help shift night owls into early birds
- Think about incorporating a self-massage and/or an autogenic exercise into your bedtime regimen. Both are described in Chapter 30, the Self-Massage and Autogenic Exercise chapter.
- Make sure you fall asleep by 10 PM. All essential processes needed to repair and reset the body happen between 10 PM and 2 AM. Sleeping between these times is key in transforming your health!

Get Nourished – Week 3

Focus on getting more love and nourishment. What do you need? Give yourself that!

It's time to make gratitude a habit
• Every day, at the first sign of the sky, give gratitude to yourself and as many people and experiences you can think of for helping you get to this moment
• Give gratitude every time you sit down to eat. Think about all the people involved in getting the food prepared before you. Give thanks to the land, the animals if involved, the farmers, those involved in transport and preparation, and maybe the person who served it. If you can't say thank you to the food for nourishing you and all involved for the care they put into serving you, the food is probably not in alignment with your health or ethical values and you should not eat it.
• Gratitude is an easy way to break up negativity before bed. If you are feeling down or worried about something, it might be time to run through your gratitude list. Self-love and gratitude toward your body can be enhanced if you do this while giving yourself a self-massage. Finish your review by listing 3 things you did well that day and one thing you will work on tomorrow.
It is time to focus on feeling happy!
• Write down a list of 40 things you absolutely love to do... that light you up... that make you feel alive! Do at least one a day!
• Here is the tricky part …. *These things should not include eating food that is not on your list of approved foods.*
• Think leisure, relaxation, love, inspiration and connection. Here are some ideas:
○ Lie on the grass and look up at the sky; talk to one of your best friends; listen to one of your favorite songs. Visit your favorite tea/coffee shop; read a not-so-educational magazine; blow bubbles; hug your pet/child. Get a facial/manicure; spend time on Pinterest; listen to a podcast. Paint; draw; write; play a musical instrument. Go to a bookstore. Go to a yoga/meditation class; shop for essential oils. Visit a museum; visit a park;

Get Nourished – Week 3 *cont.*

learn a new language. Sing; give yourself a pedicure; give yourself a massage; go to your favorite dance/Pilates/barre class. Dance; volunteer; sip a cup of tea with your grandmother or favorite neighbor, and browse inspirational quotes or make a new Pinterest board.

Get your dose of touching! .

- Massages should be a part of everyone's self-care regimen
- Massages are relaxing, detoxifying and nourishing. I wrote a post on this a while back. Look at all the benefits. See "Why Massages are Anti-Aging" in the blog section of ABeautifulRx.com.
- Consider a daily self-massage, which is described in the chapter on Self-Massage and Autogenic Exercise (Chapter 30).

Hug every day

20 seconds of contact with another living thing can promote extreme wellness, balancing hormones, stimulating oxytocin for optimal repair, combating stress and promoting whole body wellness. If human contact is just not an option, hugging an animal or a tree can be similarly effective! Remember, 20 seconds for best results!

Studies done on premature infants and animals have proven again and again the healing and nourishing power of touch. Touch helps signal to the body that it is safe and that it can rest through activation of the parasympathetic nervous system and release of the love hormone oxytocin.

Researchers have shown that touch can improve the immune system, reduce cardiovascular stress, and decrease the levels of harmful stress hormones in the body (Cohen et al., 2015).

More contact with living beings may even help you be more efficient and cognitive with physical tasks! A study was conducted at Berkeley and published in the well-respected peer reviewed journal Emotion which found that NBA basketball teams won more games when the players touched each other! (Kraus et al., 2016)

Get in touch with nature.

- Just being around trees and other living things can help wake up your immune system and promote anti-inflammatory processes, allowing your body to heal and thrive. I suggest going for a mindful walk in a place with

Get Nourished – Week 3 *cont.*

trees for 20 minutes in the early evening before dinner. Take deep belly breaths, notice all the beauty around you, naming but not judging how the air feels on your skin, the color of the sky, the trees, the grass, pointing out animals, acknowledging the wind, the temperature, the clouds and anything else you can see, hear, or feel. Try not to interpret, just notice life unfolding. Allow yourself to ride the wave of your breath and just be one with what you are experiencing. This is a sort of passive meditation and way to reconnect with the living and disconnect from the plastics and artificial materials (Maller, 2006).

- **A Mindful Walk** - Walking alone is stress relieving in and of itself. Walking in nature has even more profound effects. Results from a 2010 study in Japan showed that walking in forest environments activates the parasympathetic nervous system, promoting lower levels of cortisol, blood pressure and pulse rate (Environmental Health Medicine, 2010). Taking a walk just observing nature, breathing deeply and attempting to stay in the present moment can be an easy remedy for anxiety and feelings of disconnection.
  - During this mindful walk, you might benefit from ending your experience with a soul-connecting Kundalini mantra song. These songs are powerful, especially if you can spend time singing the mantras aloud. They are a shortcut to your soul. They can help break up chaos, help bring you love on demand, align you with your true self, and help you tap into your intuition. I encourage you to try it out. It might be helpful to listen to some of the songs suggested, find one that you feel might aid you, and sing it aloud when you get a chance. I challenge you to try it out a minimum of 3 times during this nourishing phase. If you feel it is healing and empowering, continue in the activation phase and try out a guided class. Kundalini has been one of the most essential tools in my life. It has made me less dependent and needy on outside sources of love.
  - For an extra boost of energy and a mood and health boost, when it is safe to do so, take off your shoes during your nature walk and experience the benefits of grounding.
    - Whether it be in the comfort of your front lawn, in the park, on the beach, or poolside, the moment your bare feet touch the earth there is an undeniable sensation of revived health, wellbeing, and

Get Nourished – Week 3 *cont.*

connectivity, occurring almost instantaneously.

- Contact with the earth is something many of us mistakenly do not see as helpful or necessary when it is *extremely* anti-aging and healing. Touching the earth regularly allows our body's energy to match the earth's, and restores optimal vitality to all systems, including our immune and nervous systems. This ultimately results in healthier tissues, less illness and more vitality.

  An article by Chevalier et al. in the Journal of Environmental and Public Health found emerging evidence that the benefits of contact with the earth are a part of an effective strategy against inflammation, stress, pain, poor sleep, cardiovascular disorders and other chronic conditions.

- **Grounding** can help restore much-needed **healthy electron flow**. Receiving electrons from the earth also supplies us with the necessary negative charge we need to combat these damaging molecules.

- Without a conscious connection with nature and the earth, modern life often leaves us without this healing connection, and because of this we suffer physically, emotionally and mentally.

NOTE: The Institute for Functional Medicine (IFM) did field experiments on the physiological effects of Shinrin-yoku (literally "forest bathing," or taking in the forest atmosphere) in 24 forests across Japan.

The results show that forest environments promote lower concentrations of cortisol, lower pulse rate, lower blood pressure, greater parasympathetic nerve activity, and lower sympathetic nerve activity than do city environments.

Environ Health Prev. Med.

2010 Jan;15(1): 18-26

- o Because we are more often indoors and in contact with flooring, such as wood, vinyl, carpet, sealed tile and treated marble, we are now more in tune with the chaotic frequencies of mobile phones, TVs, and the lifeless energy of synthetic materials and plastics. Shoes also prevent us from benefiting from the earth's direct current. The rubber soles completely block any conduction of natural energy into our bodies. Before shoes,

Get Nourished – Week 3 *cont.*

everyone had a healthy source of earthly contact, supplying us with extra ammunition against inflammation, and energizing the preservation of healthy tissues.

Further complicating our outdoor experience are the mobiles and other electronics we often wear on our bodies. These on-body gadgets continue to scatter the subtle, healthy energy the earth sends toward us, decreasing our immune strength.

o People receiving more direct electron flow "are more grounded." They have been shown to be less stressed, to have better muscle tension, and to have better heart rate variability. Grounding's benefits have been well documented and supported by sound evidence. We now know that regular access to grounding can promote physiologic optimization, recharging the body's lost functional capabilities. Research has shown health benefits at the molecular level. The electron flow from the earth calms restores and balances our immune system and nervous system, promoting a surge of energy-enhanced anti-oxidative activity and stimulating cardiovascular health. This healthy flow of electrons is so important to our ability to both create energy and diffuse it as harmful free radicals are produced. The electrons that the earth's contact supplies help distribute cofactors necessary for immune health, tissue regeneration, and detoxification. Studies have shown that aligning ourselves with the earth's electrical potential is beneficial for optimal health, favoring heart function, hormone regulation, sleep, balance, and better capacity to withstand stress.

So, bottom line, I encourage you to go for it! Kick off those shoes, connect, breathe, and give thanks to this free and easy restorative practice. For more on the "grounding/earthing process" read an article I wrote on my blog ABeautifulRx.com/blog.

Try out a yoga class.

During the nourishing phase I ask you to lay off the hard-core exercise and focus on what you don't usually give yourself. If you are a regular yogi, then maybe trying out a class won't be the most transformative for you and instead you should focus on other nourishing exercises, such as Pilates, barre, or a

Get Nourished – Week 3 *cont.*

different type of yoga that you know your body needs but you have never made it a point to start. For the rest of you... those who are gym rats, adrenaline junkies or those who just never considered themselves ready or "the yoga type," it's time to open your body and experience the practice of yoga.

Yoga means union with your highest self or source, so the purpose is to feel aware and connected in the mind, body and spirit so you can live in more flow, less inflammation and less suffering. The type of yoga most often practiced here in the U.S. is Raja Yoga, which includes meditation, physical poses known as asanas, and breathing practices referred to as pranayama.

Most yoga today consists of leading you through a series of these asanas and learning to coordinate them with your breath, slowing down both movement and breath to optimally stimulate the relaxation response and consequently balance the hormonal response.

Yoga helps calm the mind and nervous system to systematically bring you to a place of more awareness and consciousness. It is from consciousness that you can experience freedom from the ego (false perceptions and intellect) and ultimately experience more bliss.

The asanas help you gain awareness of the body as well, connecting your mind and your body in a way which helps you tune in to how it needs to be cared for. Practicing asanas has physical benefits as the poses help keep the muscles long and strong and the joints nourished and protected, helping protect the body from injury and promoting self-healing.

The breathing portion of the yoga practice helps nourish the cells and deep tissues with oxygen, remove impurities from the blood via better circulation, and stimulate the vagal nerve, allowing the body to work in the mode of the parasympathetic nervous system and protect you from the dangers of stress.

The meditation portion of yoga is often not the focus of mainstream yoga classes, although the synchronized breathing and movements offer some of the benefits of a formal yoga practice.

Since there are many types of yoga, it might take a while for you to connect and find the type of yoga you enjoy. I personally trained to be a Hatha Yoga teacher but found myself dedicated to an Ashtanga Yoga practice for over a decade. Today I alternate between Vinyasa, Ashtanga, and my Kundalini Yoga Practice. It took me years to know myself enough to understand which type

Get Nourished – Week 3 *cont.*

of yoga, would benefit me when.

My suggestion to you is to start your journey and experience the different types to know what suits you and your energy. I find that Ashtanga works for me when I am feeling confident in my energy and mental health (more like in the activation phase of Return to Beautiful). Vinyasa is great when I need a fusion of joy, stretching and opening of the body. Kundalini is my go-to for building love, resilience, strength and spiritual growth. Again, this is my experience but I urge you to just start, take a class this week and decide which of these practices best nourishes you today.

Practice Loving Kindness Meditation.

During this phase the focus is on getting into a place of more peace and abundance. Meditation is amazing for this. If this is your first time going through the Return to Beautiful experience, a more routine and structured practice may still not feel appropriate. Also, if you are lacking in self-love or are plagued with fear about something, meditations like the Loving Kindness Meditation could be life-changing and an amazing preparation for more formal meditative practice.

This beautiful little ritual practiced twice a day for 2 weeks could give you the strength you need to shine a little brighter and finally allow yourself to live the life you always wanted. My suggestion? Try the Loving Kindness Meditation every morning upon waking, and then before lunch. Use the Mindful Walk and Kundalini Mantra before dinner and experience the ultimate nourishing lifestyle medicine treatment. You will glow from the inside out. See Chapter 24 for a description of the Loving Kindness Meditation.

The Plan - Week 4

Overview – Week 4
- Use music to adjust healthy lifestyle rhythms
- Give love: love calls
- Use the breath
- Body Scan Relaxation Technique
- Clean out your closets: revamp

Diet - Week 4

No diet changes this week. Keep up the good work! We are still feeding the good bacteria that support better metabolism and overall health. We are also avoiding feeding the unhelpful bacteria and yeast that make it difficult for you to feel well and energized. By now you should have recycled most of your microbiome (your microbe population that your health depends on).

This said, we now want to benefit from this new population of allies, nourishing them further with foods that support them and making sure we steer clear of inflammatory foods and chemicals. By next week, your digestion should be so strong and your nutrient absorption so high that you should be able to eat less and feel much more full.

You also should be noticing a surge of energy, happiness and willpower. Your serotonin production should now be optimal, allowing you to feel more social and less dependent on quick-fix foods. You also should notice a surge in creativity and motivation.

By next week you should be able to start putting all this newfound fuel to work as you work on goals not previously possible.

Lifestyle Details - Week 4

Start making music to invigorate your mood and health.

- Upon waking, start with a song for gratitude and inspiration.
- When brushing your teeth, and getting ready, use songs for brain stimulation and creativity.
- When you need to exercise, put something on that it's impossible to sit still with.
- When driving, listen to music to combat aggression and stress.
- While at work, listen to music for concentration.
- When falling asleep after lunch, put music on to wake up the senses and that uplifts.
- *When driving home from work, put on something joyful, something that helps you connect with your source and disconnect from the ego and worries of work.*
- *After dinner, put on songs that stimulate relaxation.*
- *If you are having trouble sleeping, put on music that stimulates delta waves or contain theta waves. You can try music by Enya; nature sound recording such as rain, the ocean or wind; delta wave music; or music composed by National Sleep Foundation collaborator Frank Prince.*
- *Check out my Spotify (Jelena Ley Petkovic) for mood setting playlists.*

NOTE *Studies have shown that music has the capacity to induce the relaxation response and reduce inflammation, resulting in better health outcomes for chronically ill patients. A study in Lancet in 2010 showed significant decrease in stress hormones and inflammatory factors, such as Interleukin 6, after exposure to Mozart's music. The untapped potential of music has not been explored enough, even though eastern cultures have used sound as a medium of health restoration and healing for thousands of years.*

Music for healing from magic to medicine.

Lancet. 376(9757);1980-1

Spread the *love*!

- Call someone you care for and tell them how much they mean to you... Now that you are more full of love, it's time to share! It's important to give gratitude to the people in your life who have made you. Every time you start to feel lonely or disconnected for any reason, it's time to communicate to

Lifestyle Details - Week 4 *cont.*

others how valuable they are to you and to the world. This will light you right back up!

- Tell someone in need that they are beautiful and special. As much as it's important to show appreciation to those who are doing good work on this earth, it's also important to uplift and inspire those who are experiencing hardship or are a bit deficient in confidence. Remember, we all have the same potential and everyone has the capacity to do amazing things on this earth and we need as many people as possible to own their gifts and step up and serve. So, do your job... tell someone this week who they are... that they are divine, beautiful and special. You will heal as you heal them... love is the best medicine. Both giving and receiving work to relieve suffering and inflammation and to liberate magical powers!

- With each breath send yourself love!

NOTE According to the EWG, "Once you know the ingredients, you should avoid these seven:

- 2-butoxyethanol (or ethylene glycol monobutyl ether) and other glycol ethers
- Alkylphenol ethoxylates (some common ones are: nonyl- and octylphenol ethoxylates, or non- and octoxynols)
- Dye (companies often hide chemical information behind this word; when it's unknown, it's safer to skip it)
- Ethanolamines (common ones to look out for are: mono-, di-, and tri-ethanolamine)
- Fragrance
- Pine or citrus oil (on smoggy or high ozone days, compounds in the oils can react with ozone in the air to form the carcinogenic chemical formaldehyde)
- Quaternary ammonium compounds (look out for these: alkyl dimethyl benzyl ammonium chloride (ADBAC), benzalkonium chloride, and didecyl dimethyl benzyl ammonium chloride).

Breathe: Focus On Using Your Breath As An Ally!

- **Breathe 10 soft belly breaths before every meal.** As explained earlier, deep breathing can be a powerful tool to get you out of sympathetic stress mode and into parasympathetic relaxation mode. Relaxing before eating can be key to best digestion and promotion of mindful eating. Remember, take a slow deep breath in through your nose while filling up your belly like a balloon,

Lifestyle Details - Week 4 *cont.*

then take an equally long exhalation, letting air out of your mouth, pushing the belly button toward the spine as you release all the air. During this week, I encourage you to adopt this habit into your life.

- **When in the car, try *Alternating Nostril Breathing* or *Microcosm Breathing*.** See Chapter 25 for instructions. These methods of breathing can help you stay calm and centered even during stressful activities such as driving. They are also amazing visualization tools, helping anchor you into your body and promote awareness. If you are driving, you obviously must keep your eyes open during the activities!

I describe both exercises in Chapter 25. I hope that you use them in different situations and experience them for yourself. You may want to keep them in your toolbox long term. I personally use Alternating Nostril Breathing in traffic, and it keeps me from losing my mind! It also helps me think of traffic as a productive experience, working on my mind-body connection.

Use the Body Scan for a wind-down mindfulness practice.:

Please see Chapter 24 for instructions.

Take Another Look at Your Environment

- Revamp your cleaning closet. Cleaning supplies could be making your home a toxic hazard for you and those you love. Head to Target or your place of choice and buy green, non-toxic cleaning supplies to make your home safer to breathe in and to touch. Most conventional cleaning supplies are filled with irritants and endocrine disruptors, making health and weight difficult to manage.
- Look for products certified by the Green Seal or EcoLogo for true green standards.
- For DIY cleaning, try diluted vinegar for windows and baking soda for scrubbing. See the EWG's DIY Cleaning Guide for more recipes for cleaning specific surfaces and materials.
- The BIG no-no's are air fresheners (try essential oils), drain cleaners (better to use mechanical snakes), oven cleaners (use baking soda paste), antibacterial soap (these contain triclosan, which is toxic to reproduction, overall immunity, and health), and dusting sprays (use micro-cloth instead, requiring no dusting).

Lifestyle Details - Week 4 *cont.*

- Also, remember to pick up green laundry detergent and consider tree-free toilet paper.
- This week is also the perfect week to consider buying a high efficiency particulate air (HEPA) vacuum and air filter.
- Dust in your home can cause allergens and worse yet contain toxic chemicals. If you have any chemicals inside or outside of your home, chances are they're going to end up in the dust in your home. Cooking, animals, dry climate, construction, flame retardants, pesticides, and other chemicals all contribute to the toxic load of your dust. Once inside your home, these contaminants break down much slower than they would outside. Flame retardants found in synthetic materials, computers, TV, and furniture add an important source of indoor toxicity. Two ways to avoid these is to buy non-PBDE furniture and pillows and keep electronics in the home to a minimum and out of the bedroom. Certain people are especially sensitive to chemicals as they have poor detoxification capacity (can figure this out via testing with a Functional Medicine Practitioner) or because they are very young or elderly. For this reason, HEPA vacuums and air cleaners can be key in keeping households healthy. HEPA vacuums are better than regular vacuums at trapping small particulates, including allergens and chemicals.
- Other ways to keep toxic dust at bay is to leave shoes at the door, keep electronics dust-free, wet mop the floor, use micro-cloths to wipe furniture, choose wooden furniture over synthetics, choose products made of natural fibers, and choose stuffed furniture filled with down, wool, cotton or polyester which are less likely to use flame retardants.

Getting ready for Phase 3:

Start with a one day a week liquid cleanse.

Liquid Fast: (wait for instruction on how to use this)

8 AM: organic lemon water + PGX fiber tabs

9 AM: 12 oz. grapefruit juice with 1 tablespoon MCT oil

9 AM - Noon: Green tea and 3 glasses water

1 PM – 3 PM: 2 Cups warm chicken broth

3 PM – 5 PM: Herbal peppermint or ginger tea and 3 glasses water

5 PM – 7 PM: Green juice… sip with more tea

8 PM – 9 PM: 2 Cups chicken broth; add some olive oil, Himalayan sea salt, and other spices as desired

Chapter 19

Phase 3: Activate... Time to Get What You Want!

General Guidelines: *No Soy, Corn, Wheat, Gluten, Sugar or Alternative, Dairy, Coffee, packaged or store-bought food, or Alcohol.*
Focus On: *Whole foods, Supplements, Spices, Non-GMO, Organic For those trying to lose weight, look at the green highlighted recommended supplements.*

Overview – Week 5
- Try out the light bath
- Use the "I am loved" mantra
- Gratitude to your Higher Source
- Start Meditation practice
    - Primordial Sound Meditation
    - Kundalini Sadhana
- Diet: Make sure you see 4 colors in each meal

DIET – Week 5
Focus on getting every color on the food spectrum into your diet. There should be at least 4 different colors in each meal. The color of the plant reveals its phytonutrients or phytochemical components and therefore its protecting, repairing and healing properties. Each color group has a different set of nutrients which provide the plant with the ability to defend itself from pests and environmental stressors, remove toxins, and boost vitality. In the body, each group of phytonutrients provides essential components to enzymatic processes and immune

cascades to promote healthy circulation, detoxification, metabolism and cellular homeostasis, and to prevent cell death.

Sources of these phytonutrients come in different colors: green, yellow-orange, red, blue-purple and white. To benefit from the whole spectrum of nutrients, as each color contains different and essential phytonutrients, one must eat a variety of colors of foods. They will then work both synergistically and in parallel to keep you healthy. In general, the darker the color of the plant, fruit or vegetable, the more potent its phytonutrient concentration is.

The Plan - Week 5

Pre-Breakfast Upon Waking	• Juice of 1 organic lemon in a large 12-ounce glass of filtered water + ½ tsp Vitamin C • Take these supplements: Omega 3 (2), Vitamin D (3 drops), Resveratrol (1), Astaxanthin (2)
AM Activity Sweat	**Sweat 20 -30 minutes minimum.**
Breakfast Before 9 AM	• 3 eggs (2/3 whites and 1 yolk) + spinach or kale + veggies • or Green juice with 1 Tablespoon of MCT oil • Sip with green tea • Weight Loss (WL) supplement pack (for those wanting to lose more weight) • CLA
Between Breakfast and Lunch	• Organic Green Tea • 3 glasses of filtered water. • Supplements: Brain Vitale (memory and mental clarity) + Probiophage • 15-minute Vitamin D break. Go outside and seek the sun. The best times are 10 AM to 3 PM.
Lunch before 3: 10 Soft Belly Breaths	• Organic non-GMO plant, wild fish + rainbow of veggies • Add nuts/seeds or avocado, cabbage or broccoli every day • Garlic, onions, and spices enhance health

The Plan - Week 5 *cont.*

Lunch before 3: **10 Soft Belly** **Breaths**	• C3 curcumin • CLA
Between Lunch **and Dinner**	• Organic herbal tea (ginger or mint best) • 3 glasses of filtered water • PGX-2
PM Activity	**Walk 20 minutes – Nature preferred**
Dinner **Before 8 PM**	• Vegetable soups (vary colors) *or* Paleo Lean shake with greens, blues and reds • 1 apple or green pear (sliced) with cinnamon • WL Supplement Pack • CLA
Before Sleep	• **Melatonin 3mg (melatonin can be a part of a long-term anti-aging regimen)** • **No electronics after dinner. Relaxing music and inspirational reading.** • Sleep before 10 PM. The body is best able to detoxify and rejuvenate itself during sleep between the hours of 10 PM and 2 AM

Diet - Week 5

Breakfast	**Smoothie** Scoop of pea protein + ½ cup of berries/pineapple + 1 Cup of spinach or kale and the following: • Monday Tuesday Wednesday: Add 1 Tablespoon aloe vera, 1 Tablespoon chia seeds, and coconut oil – heals digestive tract • Thursday and Friday: Add 2 slices of avocado and 1 teaspoon flax seeds – makes smoothie rich, creamy and satisfying • Saturday and Sunday: Add a pinch of cayenne pepper – can potentially be added every day but avoid if on blood thinners or have acid reflux
Lunch	**Plant proteins and salad** • Go for non-GMO, organic proteins and a salad which ideally has all the food colors (see food color chart in Chapter 23) • For additional suggestions, see *Kitchen Sink Salad* and *Pomegranate & Goji Berry Salad* in the Recipes chapter (Chapter 28)

Dinner	**During the week:** 1 - 2 bowls of soup with herbal infusion
	
	• **Alternate colors of soup.** Each soup can host as many veggies as possible in the color assigned.
	   o **Monday** – Orange Soup
	   o **Tuesday** – White Soup
	   o **Wednesday** – Yellow Soup
	   o **Thursday** – Green Soup
	   o **Friday** – Red Soup
	
	Alternative Dinner Rotation: 2 days of Orange Soups, 2 days of Yellow Soups, 2 days of Green Soups, 1 day of Red Soup with Purple Side Dish
	
	Saturday and Sunday: Large plate of lightly sautéed or baked veggies with olive oil, ghee or coconut oil, herbs and spices. Get as many of the colors as possible onto the plate but make sure you get in the blue-purple and red foods.

Lifestyle Details - Week 5

Continue to make a habit of showing yourself daily love.
Use the breath, visualize light love protection around your whole body, listen to your body and feelings with no judgment, tell yourself you are enough and very loved.
Start each day with gratitude and a prayer of devotion
To the divine (whatever the highest power is for you, such as the universe, God, or love)
Start a serious meditation practice.
You have experienced what it's like to hold space for your meditative/mind-body practice in your day and experienced the benefits of its calming and restorative powers. A regular meditative practice will now take you to the next level of clarity, vitality and ability to activate the life and health you want.

Primordial Sound Meditation (PSM) is the most healing, nourishing, and restorative practice for me. You may already practice transcendental meditation or other meditation or have a genuine interest in them. What is important is that you start to deepen your practice with meditation, continuing the process of expanding your consciousness, detaching from the ego and improving your ability to use your higher brain functions, allowing better decision making and creativity. These practices are key to your success in reaching your highest potential, manifesting your desires, and preventing stress-related chronic disease.

Another meditative practice that is very transformative is practicing Kundalini Sadhana. This Kundalini practice is done every day at 4 AM and includes meditation, breath work, kriyas and devotional practices. It's beautiful, energizing and life-changing, especially when done over a 40+ day period.

Another transformational meditative challenge is attending a winter or summer solstice White Tantric Yoga Event.

If you are interested in expanding your practice in Kundalini, visit your local Kundalini Yoga Studio or the 3ho.org website. For more information on my Primordial Sound trainings, go to my website or find a certified instructor through the Chopra Center website.

Lifestyle Details - Week 5 *cont.*

Challenge yourself.

Pick a physical goal and work on reaching that goal at least 3 times a week. It may be to prepare for a marathon, achieve a certain weight or endurance/strength goal, or start a new/more serious yoga practice. This week, be sure to write down what small goal you are actively working on. Tell a buddy or a coach to keep you accountable.

What is a reasonable goal to work on?

Think of a goal that is specific, meaningful, action-oriented, realistic, and can be achieved in less than 3 months!

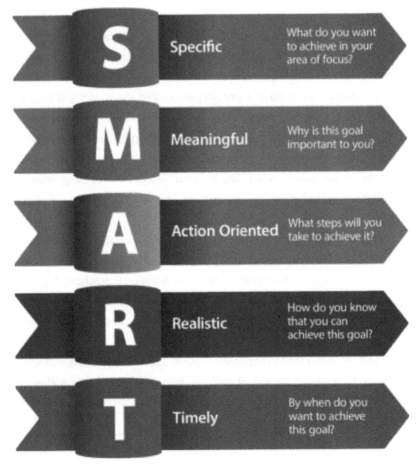

(Drucker, Peter F. The Practice of Management, 1954)

Chapter 20

Phase 3 - Week 6: The Raw Food Diet Plan

Week 6:

Attention Beautiful Beings: This is a raw food week that is optional. You should not do this if you have any digestive or thyroid concerns not managed and cleared by a medical professional. Raw diets can be hard on the stomach, and certain vegetables can be harmful to those who don't have fully functioning digestive systems or who have autoimmune diseases such as Hashimoto's thyroiditis, rheumatoid arthritis, or lupus.

If you have any concerns, please consult with your Functional Medicine Physician. Instead of the Raw Diet, you can repeat the Phase 3/Week 5 diet.

What is Raw?

- Organic, uncooked, unprocessed food, consisting mainly of fruits, vegetables, nuts, seeds, sprouted grains, raw eggs and dairy, raw meat, and raw fish.
- Food cannot be prepared at temperatures over 118 degrees (slightly warm). Anything prepared over this temperature is considered cooked and has lost some of its beneficial health properties.
- Raw food preparations can include foods that are dehydrated, sprouted, and juiced for nutrition.
- Raw milk is acceptable for most raw food advocates although dairy was adopted into the human diet less than 10,000 years

ago and may be difficult to digest for some (for humans to digest something well we need to have it in our diet for 100,000 years). Some Raw gurus also accept fermented milk while others say it is not acceptable. Fermenting food is a process in which nutrients are predigested by bacteria.

- Grains and legumes are typically not in a raw diet because they, like milk, have been part of the human diet for less than 100,000 years.
- Juicing foods is good for some, but not for those who are glucose sensitive or with certain metabolisms.
- Those who believe eating "alkaline" is the only way to stay healthy do not include meat in the raw diet.
- Those who do eat raw meat and fish need to do so with care. Our ancestors ate raw meat and therefore we can digest it and assimilating its numerous benefits. Raw meat offers more nutrients (fat, protein, vitamins, antioxidants and phytonutrients) while avoiding unhealthy sugars and toxins created during certain cooking processes.
- Eating raw means avoiding lots of unhealthy carbohydrates, since most need to be processed and cooked to eat.

Why Raw?

Some raw foodies believe cooking makes food toxic. They claim that a raw food diet can naturally assist in alleviating pain associated with inflammation such as headaches and arthritis, prevent allergies, boost immunity and memory, and prevent diabetes. Additionally, by preserving enzymes and nutrients such as protein, raw food improves digestive capabilities and helps the body to resist degenerative disease and aging.

The Nutritional Benefits of Raw Include:

- More nutrients
- More active enzymes
- More antioxidants and phytonutrients
- More protection due to free radicals
- Less rancid fats
- Less denatured proteins
- Improved digestive, immune, hormonal, and detox systems
- More suited for biological make-up

Challenges

A raw diet can make you feel worse at first because:

- Raw food may overwhelm the lymph and circulatory systems because, as cells improve function, they excrete toxins (you will later recover)
- If your biochemical requirements demand cooked food, you may not process well (more on this below)
- If you take medications and supplements that interfere with digestion, you may not feel well. Your lifestyle habits such as alcohol use, activity level, etc. can also affect your ability to digest these pure whole foods.
- You have poor digestive health (acid reflux, allergies, diseases of the gut)
- You may need distinct types of raw food... juicing, dehydrating, or sprouting. For example, some may require more juicing to feel well, while others do better with dehydrated raw food.

To prepare your gut for raw food you may need to:

In general, raw food can improve digestion due to enzyme content but eating raw food also requires more enzymes and places a larger responsibility on some other digestive processes (gastric juices, gut flora and correct bile secretion). Cooked and processed foods are much easier to digest, but lack the benefits of raw food. If you have done the detoxification and gut repair portion of this experience, you may be ready for a raw diet. This said, if you are feeling any digestive distress, fatigue or have signs of deficiency, you may want to run some tests with your Functional Medicine Practitioner.

Before you go Raw....

- You need to feel healthy. Having low energy, sleep issues, poor immunity, blood pressure issues, anxiety, depression, high cholesterol, fertility issues, or hormone imbalance may suggest there is a body imbalance that deserves your attention before you start a raw food diet.
- Get a baseline blood test and a physical. You need to know if anything about your new diet venture is worsening your health. Making sure you get a baseline will give you and your doctor a good idea where you are health-wise.
- If you don't eat any meat you may need to supplement. Ask your doctor about Vitamin B12 and selenium to start.
- Raw food requires you to be extra careful about food quality. You should eat only the highest quality fresh food to avoid food poisoning.

In summary, the raw food diet has many benefits but is not suitable for everyone and is quite difficult to maintain. I for one will incorporate as much raw food as my body will tolerate. In times of stress or sickness, or with digestive challenges, raw food might not be the right choice. What remains evident is that processed foods are never good for your health, plant fats are the ideal fats, and we should eat a variety of simple plant-dominant meals to maintain health.

How do you know which raw food diet will work best for you?

Raw food advocates say some require more a protein-based diet (including meat and fish) while others can thrive on vegetables. Knowing what is best for you requires that you take careful notice of how you feel when you eat certain food groups. You may want to do some research on your dosha (described in the chapter on Ayurvedic Lifestyle, Chapter 26), evaluate your spiritual views, and discuss with your local nutrition or Ayurveda expert if you are not sure whether a raw diet might be right for you.

Lifestyle Details - Week 6

Start the diet with a one-day liquid cleanse. Use vegetable broth this week.

Note: You can use the liquid cleanse once a week from now on to reset your metabolism, decrease inflammation, and give your digestive tract a break. Use the broth recipe in the Recipes chapter of the book (Chapter 28) for best healing power.

The Blueprint - Week 6

8 AM: Have morning super juice. Choose the juice you like best.

11 AM: Use pea protein for a mid-day smoothie

1:30 PM - 2 PM: Have a large lunch in the late afternoon. A large salad, a slice of raw bread, and half of an avocado should be standard.

4 PM: Plan a raw snack

5 PM: Dinner should a plate of raw veggies and ¼ Cup of a plant-based dip with tea

For best results

- For the most nourishing juices, use a ratio of 3 veggies to 1 fruit
- Add ginger and Matcha tea to stimulate metabolism and awaken the mind
- For smoothies, use vegan pea protein
- Use all the vegetables and sprouts you can think of in your lunch. For more savory salads, chop up veggies nice and small and let them sit in the dressing for at least 10 minutes before eating.

The Plan (Raw) - Week 6

8 AM - 9:30 AM	**Morning juice**
	Your morning juice should be sipped slowly and lovingly.
	Here is a list of my favorite options.
	Option 1: Tropical Greens (via skinny juice)
	3 kale leaves
	3 Swiss chard leaves
	1 handful dandelion greens
	1 cucumber
	1 Cup pineapple
	½ Cup lemon
	1 handful mint
	Option 2: Green Zinger (via skinny juice)
	1 handful cilantro
	4 stalks celery
	1 green apple
	½ lemon
	Option 3: Comic Love (via skinny juice)
	1 orange
	1 red bell pepper
	3 carrots
	1 lime
	Option 4: Beet Red
	2 beets
	5 radishes
	1 orange
	1 cucumber
	Option 5: Radically Perfect (via skinny juices)
	½ cup grapefruit
	1 small apple
	½ lemon
	5-6 radishes
	Dash of cinnamon

The Plan (Raw) - Week 6 *cont.*

8 AM - 9:30 AM	**Option 6: Sea Green** 　8-10 carrots 　1 orange 　1 cup spinach 　1 lemon **Option 7: PhytoBlend (via IFM, the Institute of Functional Medicine)** 　Fresh kale 　Collards 　Watercress 　Red cabbage 　Beet 　Dandelion leaves 　Parsley 　Carrots 　Pomegranate 　Berries **Option 8.　Therapeutic Super Drink (via IFM)** 　Vegetable/Fruit powder, 1-2 scoops 　Raspberry seed extract 1 Tablespoon 　Green tea extract, 1 Tablespoon 　Curcumin, 1 Tablespoon 　Pomegranate juice, 2 oz. 　Blueberry juice, 2 oz. 　Cranberry juice, 2 oz. 　Olive oil, 1 Tablespoon 　Water and stevia to taste
11 AM - Noon	**Smoothie** Pea vegan protein + 1 tsp MCT + coconut water/water + ice
2 PM - 4 PM	**Lunch** Salad (alternate varieties).　Add sprouts, onions, garlic, with nuts and seeds.

The Plan (Raw) - Week 6 *cont.*

4 PM - 6 PM	**Snack** 1 whole fruit or cup of berries with tea. Whole fruits can be apple/pear/nectarine/peach/banana.
7 PM – 8:30 PM	**Smoothie** Smoothie with green mix, 5 almonds, 1 Tablespoon flax seeds, 1 Tablespoon chia seeds, 1 cup organic unsweetened almond, hemp, hazelnut milk or other approved milk + ice Sip, alternating with tea. Make it last, then go to bed nice and early!
SPECIAL TIPS	For sugar cravings opt for adding cinnamon and/or spirulina to a veggie juice. Be sure to drink lots of tea and herbal infusions throughout the day!

Chapter 21

Understanding Phase 3

Phase 3 is meant to be a phase of health activation, sharpening mental clarity, enhancing natural beauty and expanding consciousness. It is during Phase 3 that we use the newfound health we have gained from Phases 1 and 2 to effortlessly manifest certain goals and just enjoy life.

By Phase 3 you should feel energized, have good digestion and metabolism, have predictable upbeat mood, be sleeping well, have lost unhelpful food cravings and addictions, enjoy a pain-free and lighter body, be more aware and in control of your emotions, feel empowered in your health and, yes, see yourself and the world in a more beautiful light.

If you do not feel this, it's time to further explore your ailments and possibly consult with a functional medicine practitioner as you may need more specialized support. On the other hand, if you do feel these benefits, then it's time to benefit from your newfound reset, reaching toward your dreams and missions. In Phase 3, you can continue to enhance the benefits you received in Phases 1 and 2. You can now work to take your mind, body and/or spirit to another level.

Phase 3 has two parts: a one-week guided health activation and then a more loosely woven lifestyle plan aimed to help you maintain flourishing health, prevent disease and live in flow. The one-week health activation is based on challenging the body with a more color-focused vegan raw diet to help further feed those health-enhancing microbe populations and further assist the body to detox and heal any persistent issues.

Raw plants, vegetables and fruits have, in general, higher concentrations of phytonutrients. Exceptions to this are broccoli, carrots, and tomatoes, in which cooking can enhance some of the most beneficial phytonutrients. The Food Color Chart in Chapter 23 shows the phytonutrients commonly found in different food colors and the health benefits of each.

During the activation phase, I encourage you to start an activating and loving morning ritual. Spend your days mindful of what and why you are eating, move frequently (never sit for more than an hour), and keep your evenings for relaxation and rejuvenation.

Below is a sample of an ideal lifestyle plan. This is an example of an ideal day... meaning lots of variations.

I encourage you to incorporate the most nourishing practices for you from Phases 1 and 2.

Lifestyle Overview - Phase 3

AM
1. Wake up and drink lemon water.
2. Stretch.
3. Wash hands and face.
4. Apply oil to face and massage hands and feet while taking 10 deep breaths. Visualize light entering your body with each 5-second inhalation, removing any tension and nourishing you with love. With each exhalation give thanks to as many people, things, and experiences as you can.
5. Next, practice meditation. A Mindfulness Meditation or Primordial Sound Meditation is ideal. Set aside 20 - 30 minutes. Make sure you have a designated comfortable place where you can meditate without distraction.

Lifestyle Overview - Phase 3 *cont.*

AM

6. If you need support in making meditation a part of your daily routine, seek out a meditation expert to give you a private lesson.
7. Ideally, see the sun rise as often as possible!
8. Next, exercise for 1 hour. Depending on your objectives, yoga, cardio or weight training could be appropriate here. If you don't have time to exercise, do a Shaking and Dancing Meditation, do sun salutations (5 A and 5 B), or jump rope for 10 minutes to get the body activated.
9. Have a nutrient rich, but not heavy, breakfast. I would stay away from simple carbs and sugars. Make sure you always have some protein or good fat.

Mid-Day

1. Sip teas between meals.
2. Make sure you have 3 glasses of water between meals.
3. Lunch should be your biggest meal and should be eaten before 3 PM. Make sure your plate is full of colors, spices, and a good portion of protein.

Mid-Day Tips

- Stay away from snacking unless you are a Vata (described in the chapter on Ayurvedic Lifestyle).
- Take 10 deep breaths before every meal to take you into your Parasympathetic Nervous System for the best and most relaxed digestion.
- Take a 10-minute walk after every meal.

Lifestyle Overview - Phase 3 *cont.*

Evening

1. Take a mindful walk and watch the sunset! Give gratitude to your day.
2. Meditate for 20 minutes before dinner.
3. Have a soup, vegan, or no-carb paleo dinner.
4. No electronics after dinner. Spend time listening to relaxing or uplifting music, plan for your next day, read something inspirational, or write in your journal.
5. Be in bed by 10 PM... when you don't have a hot date, important event or dance party!

Kundalini Sadhana may also be an appropriate way to get meditation and stretching into your life. Sadhana is usually practiced from 4 AM to 6:30 AM each day. The benefits have been found in the physical, mental and spiritual planes.

"The two and a half hours before dawn is called the Nectar time (Amrit Vela) for meditation because 40 breaths per breath (the greatest possible pranic energy) are available in the pre-dawn hours. The Amrit Vela is a peaceful time when the distractions and energies of the day have not battered one's body or carried one's mind away from the infinite possibilities dancing within stillness. It is a time when spiritual masters travel within their subtle bodies to bless the earth – and all those whose very presence is a blessing.

"Ideally, our aim is to maintain a meditative mind and behaviors in each moment of our lives. But early morning sadhana is the prime time and place to attune body, mind and spirit toward one's infinite nature rather than one's limitations, and toward the unity of One Self rather than divisions based on fear or anger."

– Sadhu Singh, Kundalini Yoga Miami Founder

I have practiced Kundalini at increased frequencies over the past year and I can tell you I have never experienced such a holistic healing practice. Additionally, the sense of social connection and community is priceless. The Kundalini community is non-judgmental, loving and supportive. Additionally, unlike family and other friends, the Kundalini community is always available to you, especially those centers that offer sadhana. Simply show up for a mega dose of light and love. For a long and blissful life, I recommend Kundalini to anyone. Please check out the 3Ho.org site for more information on this practice.

Chapter 22

Getting More Support

As healing and empowering as this journey may be for most readers, I know that some may crave more support. Chronic exposure to toxins, stress, sedentary lifestyle, poor food, and drugs/medications may warrant further analysis and medical care. Additionally, certain infections, diseases, autoimmune processes, and hormone alterations can also make complete healing more challenging.

The good news is, despite the gravity of your current health, the *Return to Beautiful* journey can reduce this overwhelming burden on your body, so it can focus on repairing, healing, and regulating these issues.

This said, if you are working with a physician or specialist on any medical issue, you should continue to do that during your *Return to Beautiful* experience. Additionally, if you have any suicidal thoughts or are a danger to yourself or others, ***you must seek help from a licensed professional***, and in an emergency, call the National Suicide Prevention Lifeline at 1-800-273-8255.

Finally, if you have persistent feelings, low energy, diarrhea, constipation, hot/cold intolerances, hair or skin conditions, memory loss, mood irregularities, or other unexplained symptoms, you should go see a Functional Medicine Specialist. Functional Medicine is, in my opinion, the most sophisticated medical specialty. Functional Medicine Specialists use precise methods to find the root cause of illness. They look deeply into your medical history, using laboratories to trace inflammation, allergies, deficiencies and genetic mutations to pinpoint physiological weak points that could be causing problems in the body and predisposing you to health issues.

In my experience, Functional Medicine focuses on finding diseases before they start and helping create a personalized plan to repair, strengthen and prevent further damage to the body. In clinical practice, I use many Functional Medicine protocols, especially for gut repair, hormone balance, and medical detoxification protocols.

I believe everyone challenged with a serious medical crisis should have an Institute of Functional Medicine (IFM) certified specialist on his or her care team. These experts help make sure that the whole body is considered when looking at a specific disease process. They make sure the medications are not harming the body while attacking one specific irregularity. They can work to strengthen the liver and gut, protect the brain, and improve overall immunity.

For those living in Miami who need a consultation and direction, I encourage you to contact me for a consult and some help finding the Functional Medicine support you need. In my clinic, I do food allergy testing, micronutrient testing, comprehensive hormone panels, inflammatory marker panels, pre-diabetes screening, 5-point cortisol level testing, telomere length testing, MTHFR, COMT, and celiac genetic testing, IV and vitamin boost injection therapies, and comprehensive gut health analysis. I specialize in nutritional, emotional, and environmental detoxification, hormone balance and mind- body medicine (including meditation, visualization, emotional fitness, somatic healing, and stress management tools).

For a free 15-minute consult please go to my web page ABeautifulRx.com and choose a time slot that works for you.

Part Three

Accessories to Your Healing Journey

Don't

Do It, Say It, *or* Think It

Unless It's

Healing,
Loving,
or Beautiful

Jelena Petkovic PAC MMS

Chapter 23

Food Color Charts

Orange Foods

Orange Food Compounds	Benefits	Foods
Alpha-carotene	Anti-bacterial	Apricots
Beta-carotene		Bell pepper
Beta-cryptoxanthin	Anti-cancer	Cantaloupe
Bioflavonoids		Carrots
Carotenoids	Cell protection	Mango
Curcuminoids		Nectarine
Naringenin	Immune health	Orange
		Papaya
	Reduced mortality	Persimmons
		Pumpkin
		Squash (acorn,
	Reproductive health	buttercup,
		butternut, winter)
		Sweet potato
	Skin health	Tangerines
		Turmeric root
	Source of vitamin A	Yams

Red Foods

Red Food Compounds	Benefits	Foods
Anthocyanidins	Anti-cancer	Apples
Astaxanthin		Beans (Adzuki,
Carotenoids	Anti-	Kidney, Red)
Ellagic Acid	inflammatory	Beets
Ellagitannins		Bell pepper
Fisetin	Cell protection	Blood oranges
Flavones		Cranberries
Flavonols	DNA health	Cherries
Flavan-3-ols		Grapefruit (pink)
Flavanones	Immune health	Goji berries
Luteolin		Grapes
Lycopene	Prostate health	Onions
Proanthocyanidins		Plums
Quercetin	Vascular health	Pomegranate
		Potatoes
		Radicchio
		Radishes
		Raspberries
		Rhubarb
		Rooibos tea
		Strawberries
		Sweet red peppers
		Tomato
		Watermelon

Yellow Foods

Yellow Food Compounds	Benefits	Foods
Lutein	Anti-cancer	Apple
Rutin		Asian pears
Zeaxanthin	Anti-inflammatory	Banana
		Bell peppers
		Corn
	Cell protection	Corn-on-the-cob
		Ginger root
	Cognition	Lemon
		Millet
	Eye health	Pineapple
		Potatoes
	Heart health	Starfruit
		Succotash
	Skin health	Summer squash
	Vascular health	

Green Foods

Green Food Compounds	Benefits	Foods
Catechins	Anti-cancer	Apples
Chlorogenic acid		Artichoke
Chlorophyll	Anti-	Asparagus
Epigallocatechin gallate	inflammatory	Avocado
Flavolignans		Bamboo sprouts
Folates	Brain health	Bean sprouts
Glucosinolates		Bell peppers
Hydroxytyrosol	Cell protection	Bitter melon
Indole-3-carbinol		Bok choy
Isoflavones	Skin health	Broccoli
Isothiocyanate		Broccolini
Oleocanthal	Hormone	Brussels sprouts
Oleuropein	balance	Cabbage
Phenolic diterpenes		Celery
Phytosterols	Heart health	Cucumbers
Phenols		Edamame
Phenylethylisothiocyanate	Liver health	Soybeans
Silymarin		Green beans
Sulforaphane		Green peas
Tannins		Green tea
Theaflavins		Greens (arugula,
Thearubigins		beet, chard,
Tyrosol		collards,
		dandelion, kale,
		lettuce, mustard,
		spinach, turnip)
		Limes
		Okra
		Olives
		Pears
		Snow peas
		Watercress
		Zucchini

Blue/Purple/Black Foods

Blue/Purple/Black Food Compounds	Benefits	Foods
Anthocyanidins Hydroxystilbenes Procyanidins Pterostilbene Resveratrol	Anti-cancer Anti-inflammatory Cell protection Cognitive health Heart health	Bell pepper Berries (blue, black, boysenberries, huckleberries, marionberries) Cabbage Carrots Cauliflower Eggplant Figs Grapes Kale Olives Plums Potatoes Prunes Raisins Rice (black, purple)

White/Tan/Brown Foods

White/Tan/Brown Food Compounds	Benefits	Foods
Allicin Allyl sulfides Cellulose (fiber) Lignans Lignins Sesamin Sesamol Tannins Terpenoids Theobromine	Anti-cancer Anti-microbial Cell protection Gastrointestinal health Heart health Hormone balance Liver health	Apples Applesauce Bean dips Cauliflower Cocoa Coconut Coffee Dates Garlic Ginger Jicama Legumes (chickpeas, dried beans or peas, hummus, lentils, peanuts, refried beans/low-fat) Mushrooms Nuts (almonds, cashews, pecans, walnuts) Onions Pears Sauerkraut Seeds (flax, hemp, pumpkin, sesame, sunflower) Shallots Soy Tahini Tea (black, white) Whole grains (barley, brown rice, oat, quinoa, rye, spelt, wheat)

Chapter 24

Meditations Guide

A. Mindfulness Meditation

I teach Mindfulness Based Stress Reduction (MBSR). MBSR is a means of exercising the mind to focus on the present moment. It is a tool for liberating oneself from fear, anxiety, and unhelpful rumination.

Mindfulness is the state of being fully aware and present in your life. It means you are not using emotions, anxieties, or a state of stress to react to all that you encounter as you attempt to take part in your life. Instead, you are your most authentic self and you are using your mind as your ally to enjoy and accept anything that might present itself as you move through your day.

Mindfulness Meditation is a type of meditation that helps put focus on a very specific breath touch-point over an extended period of time. While focusing attention on the breath, we are asked to not engage any of our thought process. This means that while we may recognize the presence of sounds, sensations, thoughts or emotions, we attempt not to judge them, freeing our mind to "just be" and, in a way, rest.

This rest from thought gives our brain a multitude of benefits, allowing our neuroendocrine system a nice break, and our authentic selves the ability to grow accustomed to being separated from our thoughts. Beyond a meditative exercise, mindfulness can be brought into your everyday life. Mindfulness is living in the moment and without judgment as often as possible, allowing yourself to experience life as a witness, watching and enjoying life unfold.

Why is living mindfully important?

As we age, we accumulate a series of reactions to people, places, objects and situations. Reactive habits are then programmed into our sub-consciousness psyche. We form these robot-like reactions because of what we ourselves have experienced or in reaction to the information we have been fed by others in early childhood and beyond. We use these stored reactions often because they require less time and energy than re-experiencing things authentically.

We save time and energy by skipping over what may be "unimportant," using brainless actions to move us through certain activities. Although this effort proves helpful for some things, like brushing your teeth, riding a bike, and getting to work in the morning, it often causes us to miss out on many valuable, soul-nourishing and beautiful moments.

In autopilot or pre-programed mode, we may find ourselves averse to certain situations and people, in fear of certain unfounded risks, or anxious when no certainty of discomfort or failure exists. We unconsciously rely on escape mechanisms, addictions, or bad habits to keep us from something we have no real reason to avoid. This fear, laziness, and anxiety cause us to live in a sort of safe mode, which could be the source of capped creativity, feelings of imprisonment, and possibly feelings of depression and hopelessness.

Living on autopilot means we go through much of our day without thinking, relying solely on learned and pre-wired actions to guide us. Because of this we often begin and end each day with little thought, getting dressed, driving, eating, and working without ever being in full attention of what we are doing.

I know that I was so preoccupied in my head that I used to find myself struggling to remember conversations I'd had that very day. Worse yet, on several occasions while awake and driving, I found myself at unintended destinations. As I began to experience the impact of mindless living on my overall quality of life, I questioned my friends and peers and learned that others had experienced similar bouts of confusion.

Research has shown that weak mind-body connections correlate with declining health, loss of happiness, hindered relationships, and poor concentration/productivity. Mindless living can be blamed on autopilot thinking. Living without truly experiencing and inhabiting our bodies can be linked to disorders such as overeating, anxiety, depression, ADD, heart disease, diabetes, pain, being overweight, hormone-related issues, fertility issues, lack of motivation, lack of energy, impaired ability to heal, inability to deal with stress, and skin problems. MBSR techniques will help you break free of programmed living and start taking control over your own life and destiny.

B. Detoxing Meditations

FORGIVNESS MEDITATION

My favorite two detoxifying meditations are the Forgiveness Meditation or Ho'oponopono Meditation and the Shaking and Dancing Meditation.

The Forgiveness Meditation is one learned from ancient Hawaiian traditions, allowing the healing of all suffering and stress caused by relationships in this life and past lives (if you believe in past lives). The Forgiveness Meditation allows you to clear up any negative energy, guilt, anxiety, or blame produced toward yourself or between you and another.

Without this clearance, the old habits and thought patterns may be difficult to break and will result in low self-esteem, unhelpful perceptions, and even increased likelihood of certain illness. The trick here is not to judge or blame anyone or anything for the disputes you have with yourself or with others, but to simply wish them to be dissolved and alleviated. To do this you must take responsibility for your energetic contribution and take initiative to clear any negativity from the heaviness of any relationship.

This said, when practicing forgiveness, you must also stay compassionate to yourself as you attempt to say you're sorry and say "I love you" even though your mind and emotions may experience conflicting reactions. Practicing Ho'oponopono twice a day for two minutes over two weeks should help lift and clear some barriers to flourishing health.

To Perform the Forgiveness Meditation (The Ho'oponopono process):

1. Ideally, sit where it is safe to close your eyes.
2. Envision the person you want to forgive sitting in front of you. This meditation can be used for several people in your life with whom you are not in alignment or for someone with whom you feel a hurtful disconnect… this person can even be yourself. It's important to choose a person with whom you need to dissolve tension or have poor energy with, and then focus on working on this person for a couple of weeks until the thought of this person does not impact you physically or emotionally any more. At this point, you can choose to focus on a different person if necessary.
3. Before beginning, notice where you feel the tension or pain in your body as you look at the person sitting in front of you. Rate this tension from 1 - 10 and if possible write this number down.
4. Ask the person in front of you if you can heal the relationship. If they say okay, then go on to begin the meditation.

5. Begin the meditation by visualizing and collecting a circle of light, an infinite source of healing energy or love, from above your head. Over the next slow breaths into your nose and out of your mouth, move this light into your body and out to the one with whom you want to dissolve any negativity.

6. With each slow inhalation, allow the light to enter your body and into your heart, lighting it up, filling it up with energy. Watch your heart get stronger and more luminous with each inhalation.

7. Next, with each exhalation, send that light through your body and into the person in front of you.

8. Do this 5 times before starting the mantra below.

   The Forgiveness Meditation Mantra:

   Say the following repeatedly until you feel the tension in your body dissolve or until a maximum of 3 minutes have passed. Use a timer, set for 3 minutes, when you do this.

   "I'm sorry."

   "Please forgive me."

   "Thank you."

   "I love you. I love you."

9. Try to do this twice a day for 2 weeks, or until you feel the negativity and associated tension lifted from you.

10. You can keep a journal of your experience if it helps.

SHAKING AND DANCING

I received many of my mind-body medicine skills from Dr. James Gordon's research and experience. As the founder of The Center for Mind-Body Medicine, Dr. Gordon has developed workshops to help reset people's health via experimental tools such as meditation, visualization, awareness, mindfulness and emotional detoxification techniques.

One of my favorite experiences is the Shaking and Dancing Meditation. As its title suggests, this meditation is done shaking and dancing. It is perfect for those who just can't get themselves to sit and meditate but need an emotional and physical release. I highly recommend using it as often as possible during the detoxification phase of the Return to Beautiful experience. The Shaking and Dancing Meditation is also magic for those who have little time in the morning for meditation, never mind exercise, but desire a way to get out tension, built-up energy, or emotion, and possibly to even break a sweat.

Before using this meditation, I thought the only way to get these benefits might be to go out, get drunk and dance all night *or* subject myself to some long painful cardio session. Each has certain unwanted side effects. Having an orgasm is also a great release, but its full benefits are only experienced when a whole host of situational factors are there to support it. Although self-induced orgasm may have some therapeutic benefits, I will not discuss those here. Meaningless sex has other potential physical and mental repercussions that a good Shaking and Dancing Meditation does not.

Below are the steps of the Shaking and Dancing Meditation. It has three parts: 1) Shaking, 2) Stopping and remaining still for 2 minutes, 3) Dancing. Use your phone as a timer.

1. Find some music that is not too familiar, maybe ethnic and instrumental.

A good choice is the song Dynamic Meditation by Osho.

Another good option to use is *Ang Sang Wahe Guru by Kamari and Manvir*, especially for those days you just need to get a little sweat/love/emotional detox in. I love it! It means the dynamic loving energy of the infinite source of all is dancing within my every cell. Even without the dancing, saying this alone repeatedly is a great mantra for breaking up the chaos in your life.

2. Find a safe open space.
3. Close your eyes.
4. Plant your feet shoulder-width apart. Bend your knees slightly, relax your shoulders, and breathe deeply. Then shake your body.
5. Let your body get very loose like Jell-O and move to the beat.
6. Start shaking/vibrating your body with your feet maintaining contact with the ground.
7. Feel yourself vibrate up through your feet, to your ankles, through your calves, then knees, then thighs, then hips, then abdomen, chest and heart, then your arms, shoulders, neck, jaw, brain and head.
8. Next start to follow this same pattern but start to mindfully shake out tension and whatever "un-useful garbage" is holding your body back from feeling light and free.
9. Continue to shake and vibrate out all heaviness and all confusions and imagine a wave of light coming into and feeding each area of your body as you shake and vibrate the energy of the earth from your feet up into the crown of your head and beyond. Let out any sounds your lungs feel compelled to let out... don't hold back... this is your time to let out any emotional baggage, stress or tension holding you back from your best day yet.

10. The song should last about 7 - 10 minutes.

11. When the music stops, take 2 minutes to feel the energy that was created in your body and now is pouring out of your body. Experience this in silence, just noticing what has happened after you have liberated the tension, emotions, and unhelpful energy. Notice the physical sensations, breathing, and emotions that arise. Let yourself feel whatever comes up; cry, smile, vibrate or absorb. Release anything else you need to and just witness your body and mind as they become lighter and freer.

12. Give yourself a quick "Thank you" and "I love you" before starting the last phase of the Shaking and Dancing Meditation.

13. Start your last song. This portion of the meditation is about celebration, where we focus on joy and gratitude. The song choice for this portion should inspire these feelings of bliss. This song can be any song that fills your heart and soul with love, joy and rhythm.

    One of my favorites is Three Little Birds by Bob Marley.

    Other choices to help you find your groove and let go are:

    - **Good Life**
    - **Don't Worry Be Happy**
    - **Hey Soul Sister**

You can find all my Shaking and Dancing Meditation songs on my Spotify (Jelena Ley Petkovic).

C. Nourishing Meditations

LOVING KINDNESS MEDITATION

Nourishing meditations are key when healing. I like to use nourishing meditations in Phase 2 of the Return to Beautiful experience.

Loving Kindness Meditation is a must when in need of self-love, self-compassion and support. This nourishing meditation is also ideal for increasing love, gratitude, joy, interest, and bliss in one's life. It helps increase positive emotions that contribute to higher life's satisfaction, mood, and conscious living.

Loving Kindness Meditation has also been shown to increase baseline vagal tone, or parasympathetic activity, associated with increased wellness (Kok et al., 2013). Other studies have shown that Loving Kindness Meditation can help decrease migraines, emotional tension, pain, and anger.

Like Primordial Sound Meditation, Hoge et al. showed that Loving Kindness Meditation increases telomere length, proving the meditation to be an effective anti-aging technique (2011).

For those with high Pitta energies (fire and water constitution per Ayurveda), Loving Kindness Meditation may be the best way to keep you pro-social, helpful, compassionate, empathetic, and fair. For those with low self-esteem, depressed or self-critical, Shahar et al. showed that Loving Kindness Meditation can help you build more self-love (2014).

Here is how to do Loving Kindness Meditation:

1. Get into a comfortable, cross-legged position.
2. Take a few deep breaths in your nose while filling up your belly for 5 seconds, then in your mouth while pushing your belly button toward your spine.

3. Massage the back of your neck and your shoulders. Twist your shoulders left and right and stretch out your arms overhead before resting your hands on each knee facing up.

4. Let light surround you and enter your body with every inhalation filling up your heart. With every exhalation send the light through your body and out into the world, filling up everyone in its path.

5. Repeat this mantra silently in your mind for 3 - 7 minutes:

   - *I am full of loving kindness.*
   - *I am safe from inner and outer dangers.*
   - *I am well in body and mind.*
   - *I am at ease and happy.*

6. After a few minutes, you can then direct this love and kindness to specific people or all humanity or beings:

   - *May all beings be full of loving kindness.*
   - *May all beings be safe from inner and outer dangers.*
   - *May all beings be well in body and mind.*
   - *May all beings be at ease and happy.*

7. Repeat another 3 - 7 minutes and allow the words to penetrate mind, body, soul, and the universe.

KUNDALINI MANTRA MEDITATION

Kundalini Yoga works to awaken one's personal experience and awareness through a series of "kriyas." Kriyas are a choreographed pattern of movements, sounds, pranayama (breathing), mudras (hand gestures), concentrative practices, and meditations. The kriyas help tone and waken the nervous and hormonal systems to balance the subtle energy channels in the body for optimal life experiences.

Like PSM, Kundalini's meditations use mantras. These mantras are often dedicated to the higher self, the divine, the universal, and love. These mantras help us to unite with the infinite and be nourished with love and healing powers.

One thing I specifically love about Kundalini Yoga is that many of the mantras are sung. Singing in and of itself is healing as it connects you with your heart and in turn your loving and centered soul. Practicing Kundalini has helped me find peace and love no matter what my life situation. Every time I practice it, I quickly find myself aligned with my true nature and in a state of heightened emotional fitness and awareness.

I find that practicing Kundalini in the morning allows me to flow into my day much more easily. My desires and objectives are more clearly defined, so I can manifest what is in my own heart with less effort. I also feel Kundalini helps those who practice it become more self-reliant and resilient. Like my Ashtanga Yoga and meditation practices, learning and bringing Kundalini Yoga into my life has been an invaluable gift. Now that I have these in my life, I can depend on them anywhere in the world, to bring me happiness, strength, awareness and peace.

I recommend Kundalini exercises to all during their Phase 2 nourishment phase and encourage all to attend a local Kundalini Yoga class. If classes are unavailable to you, I encourage, at the very least, incorporating Kundalini mantra songs into your day, helping you to feel connected to your true self and fueling yourself with the light of the universe. For those of you who are not ready to embrace the singing element, simply listening to the mantras with some awareness around their intention and meaning will help you transcend ego (fear, worry, memories etc.) and tap into your true power source.

D. Activating Meditations

PRIMORDIAL SOUND MEDITATION

Primordial Sound Meditation (PSM) was developed by Dr. Chopra and Dr. Simon and Indian scholars from the ancient Vedic and yoga traditions of India. PSM was revived and systematized from an ancient meditation technique tried and tested for thousands of years.

The primary purpose of PSM is to help you find out who you are, restoring wholeness and helping you not only fully heal but thrive. Like yoga, Primordial Sound Meditation aims to help unite mind, body and spirit and transcend intellect and ego to more easily access the soul and Spirit.

For me, Primordial Sound Meditation is one of the most beautiful rituals you can have in your day. The mantra must be calculated and assigned to you by a certified teacher. It is a beautiful set of words representing meaningless sounds, which replicate the sound of the vibration of the earth the moment you were passing through the birth canal or abdomen of your mother. The Primordial Sound Mantra is a perfect vehicle to higher consciousness as they are the sounds that supported you as you moved from the state of pure potentiality (inside your mother's womb) to individuality (as you emerged in the world).

There are 108 possible Mantras that can be assigned and calculated based on your birthdate, your time of birth and the location of your birth. The repetition of the Primordial Sound (PS) mantra during meditation allows you to fall more easily into the silent realm where your spirit exists, allowing maximal alignment with your true path on this earth and beyond. It is in the space between your thoughts and falls into the gap of silence where the infinite potential resides and we can break free from the destiny we were born with and activate the destiny of our hearts. The destiny of our hearts is the one where we can manifest or create as we wish, we don't suffer, and we live in more flow, experiencing a multitude of miracles and synchronicities along the way.

When you are aligned with your spirit you are in alignment with your creator, allowing better/direct lines of communication with the Universe/God/your higher self. It is when we are in this space that we can break away from old habits and thought patterns, allowing us to live a more nourishing and creative life. We can feel free and flexible, maintaining the curiosity and resilience of a child, and can easily see joy and beauty.

Once your PS mantra is given, it is to be used only during your sacred meditation time, as it will be your fastest route to the gap and your true essential nature, the one that supports your best health. The more you practice PSM, the more you will live in alignment with your true infinite nature and connect with the cosmic value of life.

PSM allows you to use the vehicle of the mantra sound to experience all dimensions of self and shift your awareness to one of witnessing. Experiencing life as a witness means you are simply observing life unfold and not experiencing it as an actor who must go through all the draining emotions of this movie called *life*. In general, the awareness and consciousness developed because of meditation means less suffering, less stress, more joy and flow, and making more creative and healing decisions. Primordial Sound Meditation, with practice, frees you from the grips of your ego, allowing you to tap into the higher realms of consciousness, feeling more connected to everyone and everything and living sustainably in grace and gratitude.

I love using PSM as my go-to meditation practice as I can practice it anywhere and for me it is the most rejuvenating. I feel that I expand as a person with each meditation. I highly suggest that everyone get his or her PS mantra and learn to properly use and apply it with a certified instructor.

I give monthly workshops in Miami and do one-on-one individual Skype guided classes for those wishing to receive their PS mantra and learn to meditate. Please request your session at ABeautifulRx.com and keep up with my courses and healing events Facebook page @AbeautifulRx by Jelena Petkovic or my Instagram @heartandsoulmedicine.

E. Basics of Formal Meditation Initiation

For those practicing Kundalini, this may seem like overkill ...so I might suggest a 20-minute formal meditation practice in the late afternoon before dinner. Consider making Primordial Sound Meditation your go-to formal practice. I find it beautiful, sacred, easy, and an excellent practice to recycle karma (past actions and experiences which cause stress and incongruence in your life) and expand consciousness.

If you don't have your Primordial Sound mantra yet, you can still benefit from the use of mantra meditation. I often coach people to use the mantra "So hum" until they get their assigned and personalized mantra.

To meditate on the mantra is simple. Just sit comfortably in an easy pose (legs crossed on the floor, back supported) or in a chair with feet placed comfortably on the floor or on a stool or books for comfort. Set your timer alarm for 20 minutes (start with 10 if new to meditation), lower your gaze, and close your eyes if you feel comfortable doing so.

- Start to repeat the mantra "So Hum" "So Hum" "So Hum" "So Hum" repeatedly.
- Slow yourself to listen and feel the mantra. Repeat it effortlessly.
- Allow it to transform as you say it; don't control it.

- Allow thoughts to come and go; gently bring attention back to the repetition of the mantra.

- Don't fight urges to sleep. It's a sign you are fatigued and need to rest. Make sure to rest appropriately and avoid eating anything or using any stimulants before meditation and sleep.

- The realm of pure awareness (consciousness and alignment with your true self) occurs when there is an absence of thought and when the mind relinquishes any attachment to time and space. It is within this realm that the benefits extend into your life, allowing you to act in more congruence with your true self and spirit. This will occur naturally, and with practice it will become more automatic with each meditation. Do not attempt to induce it! Repeat the mantra easily and effortlessly.

- Allow mental activity, then gently bring yourself back to the mantra with each distraction.

- Do not attempt to control anything and do not expect anything. Your meditation practices will mature organically and you will reap more and more benefits as your practice deepens.

There are no rules to meditation *except* to be comfortable. If you must shift your postures or legs, shift them. We don't want you to be focused on discomfort or pain when you are trying to turn your attention inward.

As you are attempting to integrate any of these beautiful practices into your life and getting a little frustrated, remember that you must make an honest commitment and stick with it. According to the Institute of Functional Medicine, transformational change takes 45 days' commitment to the positive habits. Meanwhile, negative change can be induced much more quickly, as stress and other unhelpful habits can negatively affect the body in just 7 days.

After your Return to Beautiful experience, your meditation habit might be the only habit you ever should commit to. All other healing habits may come to you with ease.

Again, a Primordial Sound Meditation course is the best way to assure confidence when integrating meditation into your life. Try finding one in your area at www.choprateachers.com or contact me on my website at ABeautifulRx.com.

F. Body Scan Techniques:

Do you have extra time in the day?

Are you feeling too wound up to sleep?

Are you having an emotional eating urge?

Do you need something to calm your nerves before an event?

A body scan can help bring you out of your head and into the awareness of your body. It is a method to sequentially bring attention and relaxation to each part of your body as you move from your toes into your head.

This is the process:

- Lie comfortably on your back on the floor or bed facing up. Get comfortable, but not so comfortable that you fall asleep.
    - o You can also practice this in a chair if lying down is not possible, making sure your feet are flat on the ground, your back is supported, and your hands are relaxed on your thighs.
- Start by concentrating on the muscles on in your feet. Contract and tighten on the inhalation, then hold the contraction and breathe for three seconds, releasing it in a dramatic fashion along with your breath.

- Take a few breaths, taking note of the area you have just consciously tensed and released. How is its position? Is there any part of it touching the ground? Clothes? How does the air feel around it? Just notice and do not try to change any sensation you notice. Just be aware of it, and then move to the next area.

- Move up to your calves and repeat the contract/tense/release sequence. Take notice of this area of your body.

- Continue this process of contracting, tensing, releasing, and noticing all the way up to your head. In sequence, focus on the thighs, the abdomen, the chest, the shoulders, the arms, the hands, the neck, the face, the eyes, and the head (contraction may not be possible here).

- At the end of your scan, envision a wave of cool blue light coming from the sky, entering the top of your head, and cleansing and calming the body as it moves down your body and into the ground.

- Finally, take 5 deep belly breaths and repeat your mantra of choice 10 times. Here are my favorites again:

    * *I Am Enough.*
    * *I Am Healthy, Happy, Whole.*
    * *I Am Light and Live to Shine.*
    * *I Am Giving, Loving and Abundant.*
    * *I am Playful, I am Powerful, I am Compassionate, I am of the Divine.*
    * *I Am Beautiful and Blissful.*
    * *I Dedicate Each Day to my Enlightenment.*
    * *I Am Perfect and will use my Intuitive Intelligence to Heal myself and the world.*

About Thinking During Your Meditation

You have not failed in your pursuit to meditate! In fact, the meditation was ultra-effective! Thinking during meditation is a method of detoxing out mental and emotional stress. After a wave of thoughts, you should become aware you stopped repeating your mantra. At the point of awareness, gently bring yourself back to the mantra. You should experience some quieting down before you experience another, smaller, wave of thoughts. Every subsequent time you are aware you are thinking and not repeating the mantra, bring yourself gently back. Over the course of your meditation, the waves of thoughts, sensations and distractions should get less and less. This is a normal course of meditation. You may notice some meditation experiences are "noisier" than others. This just means you had more stress to relieve that day! This type of information is covered in depth in a Primordial Sound Meditation course. I highly encourage everyone to find a certified instructor and empower yourself with the most beautiful self-healing/activating/anti-aging method!

Chapter 25

Breathing Exercises

A. Alternating Nostril Breathing

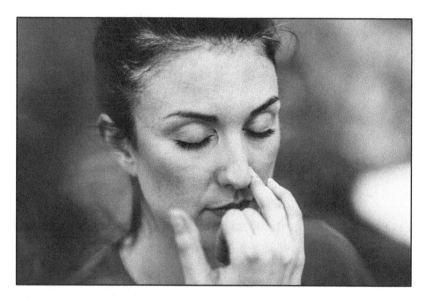

This breathing technique is referred to as pranayama by yogis… it relieves stress, rejuvenates, calms and clears the mind.

- Inhale through your right nostril over 3 long seconds while occluding your left nostril.
- Hold 3 seconds at the end of the inhalation.
- Exhale through your left nostril over 3 long seconds.
- Repeat, this time starting with the left nostril while occluding the right.
- Continue for 3 minutes.

B. Microcosmic Breathing

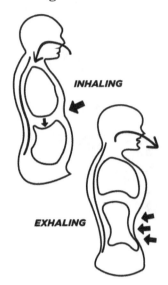

- Imagine your breath entering your body as a cool, blue, energetic light (like an ill-defined star).
- On the inhalation, imagine your breath entering through your nose down your throat and all the way down to your lower belly.
- On the exhalation, imagine your breath looping from your lower belly back up through your chest, your throat and finally out of your nose.
- Try to make as slow of an inhalation as you are comfortable with and as slow of an exhalation as possible. Try 2 to 4 second intervals.
- Push out your belly during the inhalation and pull in your abdomen toward your spine on the exhalation.
- Repeat for 2 - 5 minutes.

Even 3 - 5 slow breaths can be effective in inducing relaxation. If nothing else, try to consciously induce slow breaths throughout the day as you start to feel tension in your body.

Chapter 26

Ayurveda: Personalized Lifestyle Medicine

My advice... thrive and apply all your most valuable self-care tools as needed.

It is now time to start to personalize your lifestyle to your unique nature.

How do you do this? Although expert assistance could be of value here, my general suggestion is to learn about Ayurveda guidelines for a healthy lifestyle based on your unique energy/body constitution subtype. These subtypes are known as **doshas.**

Ayurveda, the science of life, is one of the most complete healthcare systems I have ever come across. It has deep-rooted truth to all its healing and health philosophies. In fact, Functional Medicine, the medicine that seeks to treat the cause of the disease rather than the symptom, borrows much of its wisdom from Ayurveda.

Ayurveda uses therapies that strengthen the whole body and that don't injure one area of health for the sake of another. It personalizes lifestyle guidelines, according to your underlying energy and body constitution type. It uses food, movement, rest, and lifestyle as its main prescriptions for healing and disease prevention. Ayurveda works to repair and strengthen the whole-body system, so the body can catch disease processes before they become symptomatic and prevent them from ever manifesting.

This said, not everyone's prescription is the same and depends on several patterns the person presents with at the time of consultation. An Ayurvedic physician looks first at what the patient's dosha was at birth and at how living has distorted it. The physician uses this dosha to prescribe a lifestyle regimen that will assist detoxification of unhelpful elements in the body and align the lifestyle to appropriately balance that person for optimal wellness.

The Ayurvedic system of health connects disease to three sources: physical imbalance, emotional turbulence, and spiritual disconnect. Establishing wholeness is the goal of all treatments and involves detoxification, meditation, yoga, proper diet, herbs, massage, proper sensory input (what words, sounds, and environment you expose yourself to), healthy daily routines, and regulation of emotion.

As stated previously, Ayurvedic physicians or experts typically prescribe a detoxification and healing process to correct imbalances, much like I have prescribed to you in this book. If the contents of the book have not fully helped you and you want to get further support or analysis, then I suggest consulting your Functional Medicine Practitioner, or an Ayurvedic physician, or both!

I use the wisdom of Ayurveda by uncovering patients' doshas during initial consultation. I make sure to point out certain elements of their nature, describe how their lifestyle may be adjusted to support their health goals, and make sure to include these personalized recommendations in their health maintenance programs.

The Doshas

The three major doshas are known as Vata, Pitta and Kapha. Although we all possess elements of all three doshas, knowing which dosha you are dominant in can help you know how to best balance your lifestyle to keep yourself healthy. To find out what your dosha is, please visit the Chopra Center's quiz at:

https://store.chopra.com/dosha-quiz.

Ayurvedic healers have been personalizing lifestyle medicine for centuries. Long-term health maintenance means respecting your own dosha, or underlying core energy. Once issues of toxicity and lack of nourishment are addressed, it's time to follow a lifestyle which best balances you. Understanding your dosha is key to helping you know how to best keep yourself fit and strong, and how to best prevent disease.

Although full exploration of the doshas (mind-body constitutions) will be limited in this book, I want to give you enough information to make you more aware of your core energetic being and how to best care for yourself once you have worked so hard to reset your mind, digestion and habits to a place where flourishing health is possible.

There are three main mind-body constitutions: Vata (air and space qualities), Pitta (fire and water qualities) and Kapha (water and earth qualities). Most people are dominant in one mind-body constitution with some smaller degree of another or two. As stated previously, these mind-body patterns are determined at conception but life experiences influence the current state. You can understand which mind-body subtype you are by matching your qualities to the most common qualities of each dosha.

Dosha Tendencies

Vatas resemble the wind. They are cold, light, dry, irregular, mobile, quick and changeable. When Vatas are in balance they are energetic, creative, adaptable, show initiative, are good communicators, and are spontaneous. When Vatas are imbalanced they are anxious, they worry, they are inconsistent, they have insomnia, and they suffer constipation, gas, and bloating.

Pittas resemble a flame. They are hot, light, intense, penetrating, pungent, sharp, acidic and moist. Their build is medium. They have a strong digestion, warm body temp, and a sharp intellect. They are direct and precise, follow routines, and are courageous. When Pittas are in balance they are bright, warm, good at making decisions, leaders, and have strong digestion. When Pittas are out of balance they are angry, irritable, critical, judgmental, aggressive, and suffer from skin rashes, inflammation and indigestion.

Kaphas resemble natural solid materials on this earth and in general are heavyset, have smooth skin and thick hair, sleep well, move slow, have good stamina, are easygoing, are methodical and thoughtful, and enjoy routine. When Kaphas are balanced, they are steady, consistent, loyal, strong, supportive, content and calm. When Kaphas are imbalanced they are dull, inert, needy, attached, congested, overweight, complacent, and overly protective.

Understanding your dosha will help you set yourself with a successful lifestyle, one that balances your nature. Additionally, knowing your dosha will make it simpler for you to direct your vision, goals and expectations.

Dosha Balancing Remedies

Vatas need rest, steady nourishment, regularity, light, quiet time, and meditation. They need to take warm baths, and avoid mental strain, stimulants, multitasking and overstimulation.

Pittas need moderation, calm, attention to leisure, exposure to natural beauty and outdoors, long evenings to wind down, and to avoid stimulation and strenuous activity. They need meals that are balanced in flavors and served only three times a day. Pitta pacifying foods are sweet, bitter and astringent.

Kaphas need exercise, weight control, stimulation, exposure to variety, and warm and dry environments. A Kapha pacifying diet includes pungently bitter and astringent foods that are dry and spicy. Kaphas do well with regular fasting. Drinking warm liquids and exercising every day keeps them in balance. Luxurious lifestyles do not serve them.

Studies have shown that doshas tend to have specific genes and physiologic functions which require different types of self-care and nutrition!

Chapter 27

Eating for Flourishing Health

Once you have completed the Return to Beautiful Healing experience, you may feel better than you ever have in your life. This does not mean you are immune or resistant to the constant threat of poor lifestyle and food choices.

To maintain your health, you must have a plan to keep your body protected, nourished and functioning its most efficiently. As we age our body is challenged at an increased rate due to lack of intrinsic resources and heavier burden of toxins. We also need the highest nutrient foods to keep up with all the repair our aging bodies are faced with. All this said, eating for flourishing requires good basic education on what and how to eat for sustainable health. Nothing disappoints me more than when a patient who has fully regained vibrant health returns to old eating habits and must again start their healing from the same lower vibrational start point.

The ideal is that you continue to learn about your body and optimize on your newfound vitality to a point at which you feel better and better at an older and older age. To do this, learning how to eat for flourishing health is essential!

What to Eat

Eating organic and non-GMO foods is ideal because you are reducing the overall toxic load on your body. Additionally, those foods that are organic, locally grown, free-range and wild are the healthiest food choices. The animal products are more likely to be treated well and therefore contain fewer hormones and antibiotics.

The local products are more likely to be less processed, less sprayed, picked ripest, and richer in vitamins.

However, I know that being picky about your food results in more expensive food bills, straining many households' finances. For this reason, I propose a middle ground… at least avoid the conventionally grown produce known as the "Dirty Dozen." The Dirty Dozen are the most heavily sprayed produce, making them the most harmful for your health. They are:

- Apples
- Peaches
- Nectarines
- Strawberries179
- Grapes
- Celery
- Spinach
- Sweet bell peppers
- Cucumbers
- Cherry tomatoes
- Snap peas
- Potatoes

In addition, if I cannot peel the skin off a vegetable or fruit before I eat it, I buy it organic.

For more on the safest food choices, check the environmental working group at EWG.org.

In terms of animal products, I encourage you to eat meat only as needed by your constitution and lifestyle. I encourage you to eat animals with dignity and respect, and understand that that animal's life was taken so that you can live and do great things. I propose that you ask yourself prior to eating meat if it is necessary for you to thrive. Is this animal serving you so that you may fulfill your highest purpose?

If the answer is yes, look at the meat and make sure you understood where it came from, and again ask yourself a question.... Was this animal raised with the dignity and health that I would want to incorporate into my body? If yes, then proceed to say your gratitude to the animal and the world and vow to make its sacrifice worth you eating it.

I believe this is the only way to eat animal products... with consciousness and respect. There is way too much violence, pollution, and poorly spent resources in the meat industry. We need to think rationally about eating meat. We eat way too much of it and this is not sustainable for health or the fight on hunger.

To create a world in which peace is possible, there is enough food for all, and we are combating disease, we need to work together and make more rational decisions. I do believe meat and animal products can be healing for some and necessary for health for others, but what is happening now is just pure abuse to these beautiful beings.

The Functional Rules of Eating: How and When to Eat

To maintain health, and attempt to create ideal meal experiences, follow these rules of mindful eating commonly taught at the Chopra Center:

1. Keep every meal savory by ensuring it contains all six tastes: bitter, pungent, sour, astringent, salty, and sweet.
    -   **Bitter:** Found in foods such as squash, broccoli, greens, spinach, kale, and Brussels sprouts.
    -   **Pungent:** Found in spices and garnishes such as pepper, cayenne, ginger, garlic, onion, leeks, chilies, basil, thyme, mustard, and horseradish.

- **Sour**: Found in fruits, citrus, berries, tomatoes, yogurt, vinegar, pickles, and fermented foods.
- **Astringent:** Found in foods such as beans, legumes, lentils, tea, cranberries, pomegranate, apples, and peas.
- **Salty**: Found in spice and foods, such as Himalayan sea salt, seaweed, fish, meat, and soy sauce.
- **Sweet:** Found in nuts, oils, fruits, starchy vegetables, animal products, and sweeteners (honey, agave, sugar, stevia).

2. Bitter and pungent spices are best to help protect you from toxicity.
3. Depending on your dominant dosha, or energy type, you may want to increase certain tastes and decrease others. Some examples of this are the following:

- Vatas should avoid too much pungent, bitter and astringent, and add some sour and sweet to their diets to keep in balance.
- Pittas should avoid too much pungent, sour and salty, and add a bit of sweet, bitter and astringent.
- Kaphas should avoid sweets, sour and salty, preferably choosing pungent, bitter and astringent.

4. Eat only when you can sit down and relax.
5. Chew each bite on average 30 times and at a moderate pace.
6. Eat without distraction, avoiding watching TV or electronic devices.
7. Eat only while hungry.
8. Eat until you are 2/3 full.
9. Eat your largest meal at lunch.
10. To promote better digestion, reduce cold food and beverages, sip hot water or green tea, and use ginger and herbs.
11. Use supplements.

- Unfortunately, the topsoil in this country is so nutrient poor that even those who eat a strictly organic and local diet will not receive all the protective nutrients they need from food alone.
- To maintain health, a high-grade multivitamin can prevent common deficiencies leading to increased susceptibility to infection and disarray.
- Other supplements that should be taken long-term include Omega 3, Vitamin D, and some form of intermittent pre/probiotics.
  - We are rarely able to receive sufficient Omega 3 from food sources alone. Vitamin D is also vital to both the immune and the nervous systems. Vitamin D is made primarily in the skin and requires UVB sun exposure. Those who live in cooler and less sunny climates, work indoors all day, or have darker skin types are all at high risk of deficiency. For these reasons Omega 3 and Vitamin D supplementation can be considered standard in long-term health maintenance.

Chapter 28

Recipes

Kitchen Sink Salad

2 handfuls rocket or your favorite leaf
¼ cucumber, chopped finely
½ celery stick, chopped finely
2 spring onions, chopped
½ Cup mango, chopped
½ or whole avocado

Create some "sprinkle pots" full of nuts, seeds, dried fruit and anything else you want to top your salad with. My usual go-to's are pumpkin seeds, sunflower seeds, berries and hemp seeds (http://www.rawliving.eu/catalogsearch/result/?q=hemp+seeds).

Pomegranate and Goji Berry Salad

2 handfuls of rocket leaves

2-inch chunks cucumber (sliced into thin rounds, stacked on top of each other, and sliced into strips)

½ avocado, cubed

¼ red pepper, chopped into small pieces

2 florets broccoli, chopped into super-fine pieces

1 handful goji berries

1 handful pumpkin seeds

1-2 handfuls pomegranate seeds

1 small handful shelled hemp seeds

In a medium bowl, combine all ingredients; add Dressing (recipe below) and toss well.

Dressing

2 Tablespoons cold-pressed olive oil

1 Tablespoon apple cider vinegar

1 Tablespoon lemon juice

1 garlic clove, crushed

¼ teaspoon turmeric

Pinch black pepper

In a small bowl, combine all ingredients and mix well.

Vegetarian Broth

Key ingredients:
- Onions
- Shallots
- Garlic
- Celery
- Fennel
- Seaweed: Kelp or preferred (check with doctor if you have thyroid issues)
- Nettles
- Ghee *or* Extra virgin olive oil
- Himalayan sea salt
- Unbleached soup sock

Add a variety of vegetables, such as:
- Potatoes
- Turnips
- Celery
- Zucchini
- Rutabagas
- Parsnips
- Carrots
- Beets
- Zucchini
- Squash
- Cabbage

Additional herbs (as many as you like, to taste):

- Parsley
- Oregano
- Basil
- Thyme
- Bay Leaves
- Whole Chiles

1. Peel all vegetables. Keep both the peeled vegetables and the peels. You will use all of them in the broth.
2. Sauté onions, shallots, and 2 cloves of garlic (chopped) in ghee or extra virgin olive oil until soft and clear. Add a touch of Himalayan sea salt.
3. Place the vegetable peels in the soup sock.
4. Chop the vegetables, and put them aside. Later, you will add them to the soup.
5. Put celery, fennel, seaweed, and the nettles into a pot. Add filtered water until the pot is 2/3 full. Simmer until tender for 10 minutes.
6. Add the herbs and the soup sock to the pot. Cook for an additional 30 minutes until the peels are tender.
7. Add all the chopped veggies you want into your soup and cook until tender.
8. Remove the soup sock and discard the vegetable peels. Your soup will contain most or all the nutrients from the vegetable peels.

Bone Broth Base

The best bones are from grass-fed and organic cattle and poultry and from wild fish. Marrow bones can be extra nourishing to your immune system.

Key ingredients:
- 3 lbs. bones (I use roasted chicken, but you can use raw)
- Ghee
- Coconut oil
- 1 handful cloves
- 1 handful fennel seeds
- 1 lb. baby carrots
- 4 bulbs garlic, peeled
- 4 onions, chopped or sliced
- 1 bunch parsley, whole or chopped
- 1 bunch cilantro, whole or chopped
- 1 bunch celery, whole or chopped
- 1 Cup dulse flakes
- 1 knot kombu, whole
- 3-inch burdock root, whole or chopped
- 8-inch ginger root, whole
- ¼ lb. shitake mushrooms (anti-candida), whole or chopped
- 1 Cup raw apple cider vinegar
- 2 Cups lemongrass dried or 3 large lemongrass sticks
- Cumin, garlic powder, turmeric, Himalayan sea salt

1. Begin by lightly sautéing onions, fennel, cloves and garlic with chicken bones in the bottom of soup pot with ghee and coconut oil.

183

2. Add bones, ½ of the raw apple cider vinegar, and the root veggies (carrots, ginger, burdock).
3. Fill pot with water and let simmer for a few minutes.
4. Add in celery, dulse, kombu, cilantro, parsley, and lemongrass.
5. Cook on low/med for 6 hours covered, adding water as you go.
6. Season with sea salt, cumin, turmeric, garlic powder, and the remaining apple cider vinegar.
7. Add your mushrooms. Cook for 6 more hours on low/med, adding water to keep it from evaporating.
8. Simmer this soup for 24 hours.
9. When done, let cool, then skim out any bone fragments and fat on top.

In your blender, blend up the rest of the bits and pieces of veggies and spices with broth, then strain so that you are left with a clear brown broth.

Taste the broth and season to your liking.

It will be good for about a week in the fridge.

Why Bone Broth?

Bone broth is (a) mineral rich, (b) anti-inflammatory, (c) immune enhancing, and (d) contains gelatin and collagen like properties to help with gut soothing and skin/tissue/joint health.

Chapter 29

Kundalini Songs: Instant Peace, Healing, Connection

Kundalini Songs

There is no quicker way to change your energy state or mood than with music. Kundalini mantras have been sung for thousands of years. They are sung in Sanskrit, a language which neurolinguistically activates the brain and nervous system like no other language. They help you connect more quickly with your source powers. These mantra songs are some of my favorites. Use them to strengthen your spiritual connection. I often use them in my workshops to help remove mental blocks, to cultivate a connection to the higher self and intuition, and to help people find love within themselves. You can find them all on my "Spiral of Light" playlist on Spotify by Jelena Ley Petkovic.

For Peace and Rest

Antarjaamee – Try Ajeet Kaur's version

The Mantra:

Antarjaamee purakh bidhaatae sardhaa man kee poorae

Nanak das eihai sukh maagai mo kau kar santan kee dhoorae

Translation:

Knower of hearts, architect of destiny, the one who fulfills the longing of this mind.

Servant Nanak asks for this peace. Let me be the dust at the feet of the saints.

The words can be chanted before sleep to bring peace and ease to your rest. It turns our minds toward the infinite before we go unconscious for sleep, or for the final sleep of dying, allowing our minds to be in an ideal state of peace for rest and rejuvenation.

Listen to this song to give gratitude to your earthly experience but also to let go of that which doesn't serve you, and make space for new beginnings and higher love and vibration. I love this as a cleansing and connecting tool. Whenever I am upset about something silly, I play this to connect with my heart, give gratitude for all I have, and open my heart for more understanding and wisdom.

For protection: Release of fear

Aad Guray Nameh – Try Jai-jagdeesh version or Nirinjan Kaur Khalsa

The Mantra:

Aad Guray Nameh, Jugaad Guray Nameh, Sat Guray Nameh, Siri Guru Devay Nameh

Translation:

I bow to the primal Guru, I bow to the truth that has existed throughout the ages, I bow to True Wisdom, I bow to the Great Divine Wisdom

This is a mantra of protection and is recited to invoke the protective energy of the universe.

Today we listen/chant   for connection and the higher energy we have made space for. This will give us safety as we move toward the things we are meant for and the life we are meant to live. I use this mantra song to gain trust in my path, help me feel safe, and prepare me to listen to my intuition (my gut and my heart) in the decisions I need to make.

If you can just take a break to sit somewhere with your eyes closed, try putting your hands over your heart and singing along, or just listen. At the end of the song, ask yourself any important questions you have been pondering and *wait*... until your heart answers (my favorite way to get deep heartfelt insight).

To transcend old life patterns, move past obstacles with ease
Mul Mantra – Try Snatam Kaur version
<u>**The Mantra:**</u>

Ek ong kaar, sat naam, karataa purakh, nirbho, nirvair

Akaal moorat, ajoonee, saibhang, gur prasaad. Jap!

Aad such, jugaad such, Hai bhee such, Naanak hosee bhee such.

<u>**Translation:**</u>

One Creator. Truth is His name. Doer of everything. Fearless, Revengeless, Undying, Unborn, Self-illuminated, The Guru's gift, Meditate!

True in the beginning. True through all the ages. True even now.

"The Mul Mantra is a fate killer. It removes the fate and changes the destiny to complete prosperity." Yogi Bhajan

Today we chant to help transcend all obstacles, get the blessing of the universe to release karma, and move toward abundance and prosperity.

Want to rewire your brain for more creativity, breaking free of past life and thought patterns and addictions? I love the Mul Mantra for creating more possibilities. Remember the talk about neuroplasticity? This is great for this, breaking up patterns that don't serve us and instead finding new hope and a brighter future.

To release negativity, connect with intuition, accelerate manifestations

Ek Ong Kar Sat Gur Prasad – Jai Jagdeesh

Expand into intuitive knowing.

The Mantra:

Ek Ong Kar Sat Gur Prasad.

Translation:

There is one Creator of all Creation. All is a blessing of the One Creator. This realization comes through Guru's Grace.

One of the most sacred of all mantras, it should be treated with care and respect. It is often recommended that you chant either the Mul Mantra or the mantra "Aad Guray Nameh, Jugaad Guray Nameh, Sat Guray Nameh, Siri Guru Devay Nameh" to create a sacred space and energy around you before you even touch this mantra.

This mantra is the only Kundalini mantra that places you in such alignment with the divine that it comes with a warning. After you chant this mantra, all thoughts are a risk of manifestation, meaning that you *must* watch your thoughts and actions after chanting it.

Its other quality is that it is extremely effective in reversing negativity into positivity. Use it when you feel that your happiness and positivity are being subtly derailed by negativity.

If you are stuck in life, drowning in negative thoughts or fear, sing this after the Mul Mantra. Today, as you sing this song, you take ownership over the power within you to create your most beautiful life, for yourself and for the world.

Sing this song whenever you need to break from negativity to positivity and connect with your intuition or your higher self. With this song, we bring ourselves to a place where we can manifest anything we want.

Again, be careful what you think about after listening to this song... be in a gentle, compassionate and careful mindset.

For healing yourself and others

Guru Ram Das (Miracle Meditation) – Try Ajeet Kaur or Mirabai Ceiba's version

<u>**The Mantra:**</u>

Guru Guru Wahe Guru, Guru Ram Das Guru.

<u>**Translation:**</u>

To transcend from the darkness and into the light.

This is the mantra of miracles and healing.

As you listen/sing this, use light to scan and heal yourself and others. I love scanning my body as I sing this song, clearing out anything in the way of my own healing, and then scanning the bodies of all those I love to help clear out anything that could be holding them back from their own healing.

Chapter 30

Self-Healing: Massage and Autogenic Hypnosis

Self-Massage

People assume that the only way to get a massage is from a licensed masseuse and therefore it is only for those who can afford this luxury. In Eastern medicine practices, such as Ayurveda, massage is essential in keeping the tissues and nervous system healthy. A regular habit of massaging your body can be the ultimate anti-aging and preventative disease tool, and all it takes is 7 - 10 minutes every morning or evening to keep you refreshed, assist your lymphatic system to remove toxins, and get your body out of stress mode. For those who are super busy, nighttime self-massage can be fantastic for calming you down after a super busy day and prepare you for a fantastic night of sleep.

- Self-massage is super easy. If you have dry skin and are easily cold, use a rich oil such as sesame or avocado oil. If you have oily skin and are often sweaty, try oil such as coconut oil (anti-inflammatory and antibacterial). If you have very thick skin, you may want to try mustard seed oil on the body and hazelnut oil on the face.

- Sit on the floor. If you have long hair, tie your hair up off your neck.

- Start without oil and start massaging your temples and the front of your scalp in small circular motions. Move toward the back of your head using all your fingers to firmly apply pressure and alleviate any scalp pressure or pain. Go to the back of your neck and start to apply deep pressure, first with all fingers looking for sore spots, and when you can locate them start to gently apply circular pressure to that area, stretching your neck left and right while opening up that area.

- Next, take a bit of the oil and start to work down your neck and to your shoulders. Pinch and place pressure first to find the sore areas and then work through those areas with the circular motion.
- Next, start to work down the shoulders to the arms and find the points between the muscles and follow that path, gently massaging in small circular motions mostly with your thumb, index and middle finger. Again, if you find any sensitive areas, stay in that area and massage through that area with the gentle but firm circular motion.
- Next, place more oil into your hands, rub your hands together, and then move to work on your wrists and hands. It's a good idea to first break through the initial tension with the sequential pinching of each area of the wrist, hand, and fingers. Play special attention to the area below the thumb on your palm and don't forget to put pressure around each nail.
- Next, apply more oil and move to the anterior neck and chest and, if applicable, the breasts. Large, gentle circular motions will help release tension. Make sure to pay attention to the underarm area where some of the most important lymphatic glands are located. This is a great way to get to know this part of your body and be aware of any early changes that may occur.
- Next, add more oil and move to your abdomen and make sure to massage in a circular motion starting at the outer aspects of your abdomen and then moving toward the middle around your belly button. Work this area twice over, and if you have

any problems with constipation I recommend continuing until you feel you've reduced any areas of tension or firmness. In the case of constipation, it's always a good idea to massage in a horizontal U shape, starting at the left upper corner, moving across your upper abdomen, down the right lateral abdomen and across the inferior abdomen toward your lower left corner. Another motion after the U shape that could be beneficial is to then start at the upper abdomen and move toward the bottom half of your abdomen, moving from the right side to the left in a linear fashion.

- Next, with a fresh squeeze of oil, move from your feet up to your thigh if massaging in the morning and from the thigh toward the feet at night. The direction we massage the legs depends on if we want to increase our energy (in the morning) or decrease our energy (at night). If massaging in the evening, for example, start at the top of one of your legs, massaging the thigh, then move on to the calf and shin and then the foot. After you complete one leg, move to the other leg. The best technique in these areas is to find a space between the muscles and move in a small circular pattern between the muscles and then massage in a larger, more global fashion up and down the leg. In the feet, it's beneficial to use your thumb and apply deep pressure and move in small motions to release any tension before moving to the next area along each area of the foot. Do not forget to squeeze and gently pull the toes. Before finishing make sure you flex and point each foot and use a few motions to refresh each foot. Stretch out your legs and finish with any last stretches before moving on to the rest of your day or moving on to bed.

- Watch the video of self-massage at:
  ABeautifulRx.com/ReturnToBeautifulresources.

Autogenic Exercise

Autogenic sleep training is the exercise of repeating phrases to the body suggestive of certain physiological processes that occur naturally while you are falling asleep. Repeat each of these phrases silently to yourself until your drift into sleep.

- My legs are heavy and I am at peace (6 times).
- My arms are warm and I am at peace (6 times).
- My heartbeat is calm and strong and I am at peace. (6 times).
- My breathing is calm and relaxed and I am at peace. (6 times).
- My abdomen radiates warmth and I am at peace. (6 times).
- My forehead is pleasantly cool and I am at peace. (6 times).

Recommendations by the Institute of Functional Medicine for better sleep include:

- Avoid alcohol 3 hours before sleep
- Avoid caffeine after Noon
- Avoid decongestants and cold medicines at night
- Avoid exercise after 6 PM
- Avoid the news or other media during dinner
- Avoid naps after noon
- Avoid naps longer than 45 minutes
- Avoid heavy, spicy meals at dinner
- Avoid eating after dinner
- Avoid drinking more than 4 - 8 ounces before sleep
- Take a hot salt/aromatherapy bath before sleep. A warm shower can help too.
- Lavender oil and Epsom salts in your bath will promote relaxation, and decrease cortisol stress hormone before sleep
- Listen to relating music and/or read inspirational but calming reading material before sleep

- When attempting to sleep, don't stay in bed more than 30 minutes attempting to do so. It is better to get out of bed and return to try again.
- Make sure windows are covered well and early light cannot creep into your room and interrupt your sleep
- Close windows if noise is likely to wake you up early
- Sleep in a cool environment
- Use hypo allergenic pillows
- Avoid waterbeds and the use of electric fields near your bed
- For those who sleep on their side, consider using a side pillow, hugging pillow and putting between knees for better spinal alignment
- Sleep on the best linens that you can afford
- For those struggling to fall asleep consider taking the following supplements:
  o Melatonin: 1 - 5 mg to fall asleep or 5 - 20 mg time released to stay asleep
  o 5HTP: 50 - 300 mg 1 hour before bedtime
  o Taurine: 500 - 2000 mg 1 hour before bedtime
  o Magnesium/Calcium: 250 - 500 mg or Magnesium citrate or glycinate 400 - 800 at bedtime
  o An herbal tea habit before bedtime can help support relaxation before bed. Try lemon balm or passion flower.
- Morning Blue light therapy or 10,000 lix bright light exposure upon waking can help shift night owls into early birds
- Think about incorporating a self-massage into your bedtime regimen
- Consider an autogenic exercise

- Make sure to fall asleep by 10 PM. The best time to repair and reset the body is between 10 PM and 2 AM. Don't miss out on this prime rejuvenating time.

Chapter 31

Healing Journey Resources

A. Your Food Shopping List

Starter Kit

PGX (2-4 capsules 2 - 3 times a day)

Organic green tea
Organic detox tea
Organic peppermint tea

Organic ground flax seeds
Organic chia seeds
Organic pomegranate juice/tart cherry juice (phase 2)
Organic apple sauce (phase 2)
Organic almond butter (if desired)

Organic cold-pressed olive oil
Organic flax oil (salads)
Organic coconut oil (high cooking)
Organic ghee (high cooking)
MCT (coconut oil)

Organic kimchi: 1 tbsp. per day to ¼ cup per day (Phase 2)
Green food supplement: to use if you don't get in your detox
veggies or are not eating enough greens

Stevia: as needed for a drop of sweetness

Himalayan sea salt: no other form of salt to be used

Apple cider vinegar

Other Groceries – Alternate

Spinach (3 Cups)

Kale (2 Cups)

Cilantro (3 Tablespoons)

Parsley (3 Tablespoons)

Broccoli (1 Cup)

Brussels sprouts (1 Cup)

Celery (2 stalks)

Cabbage (2 Cup)

Seaweed (¼ Cup)

Mushrooms (½ Cup)

Bok choy (½ Cup)

Organic lemons

Organic apples (1 - 2)

Organic apricots (1 - 2)

Organic cucumbers (1)

Organic carrots (1 - 2 large)

Broccoli (1 Cup)

Carrots (1 Cup)

Cauliflower (1 Cup)

Sweet potatoes or regular potatoes with skin (1)

Cooked lima beans (1 Cup)

Onions

Garlic

Ginger

Milk alternatives: Unsweetened organic
- Almond milk
- Coconut milk
- Rice milk
- Hemp milk

Condiments
- Rice vinegar
- Red wine vinegar
- Organic apple cider vinegar

Nuts / Seeds
- Raw almonds, walnuts, pumpkin seeds (add to salads, do not snack)

Allowed carbohydrates (best for lunch)
- Potatoes, sweet and white
- Organic brown rice (frozen)
- Organic white
- Lentils
- Split peas
- Quinoa
- Gluten-free oats
- White beans

Organic produce
- Fruits (apples, pears, berries ideal) and all veggies
- Organic herbs: mint, parsley, basil, dill, thyme, sage, rosemary

Proteins: grass fed, organic, non-GMO fed / wild for fish
- Ground turkey
- Lamb chops
- Chicken breast
- Wild salmon
- Wild flounder

B. Journaling Guide

Yes or No

Did you sleep well last night?

Did you have any time to relax?

Did you get any exercise in?

Did you get to stretch?

Did you get healthy communication in?

How did you alleviate stress?

Some questions to ponder

What was your overall impression of today?

What did you do well? (that made you proud or happy)

What is one thing you would like to improve on?

Write down which of these emotions best describe your day.

Energetic	Balanced	Relaxed
Optimistic	Compassionate	Sad
Loving	Creative	Frustrated
Playful	Aware	Upset
Happy	Grateful	Worried
Forgiving	Honest	Fearful
Expressive	Joyful	Stressed
Authentic	Self-accepting	Anxious
Appreciative	Solution Oriented	Depressed

How do you think your diet affected your overall mood? What else affected you disposition?

C. Supplement List

The following supplements are recommended to improve your Return to Beautiful experience. All of you who have purchased the book get a 15% VIP discount on all products bought at ABeautifulRx.com/shop.

If you are under the care of a physician, please get all supplements cleared as appropriate for your condition.

Phase 1: All to be used as directed.
- Prebiotic Focus: Feed your liver and feed your gut
- Paleo Cleanse Protein Powder
- Paleo Cleanse Supplement pack (Digestive Enzymes, BCAAS)
- Vitamin C Bio Fizz
- Vitamin D
- Omega 3
- PGX
- Curcumin: up to 400 - 600 mg 3 times a day
- Colon Rx: Ayurvedic

Phase 2: Accelerate gut health and restoration. Take as directed.
- Probiotics: Probiophage
- GI Repair

Phase 3: All optional and to be used as directed).
- WL supplement Pack
- Brain Vitale
- Resveratrol
- CLA
- Curcumin (turmeric)
- Melatonin

.

D. Wellness Checklist

Week# _____

Lifestyle Homework _____

Wellness Activity	Mon	Tue	Wed	Thur	Fri	Sat	Sun
Visioning							
Inversion							
Acupressure							
Stretch							
Journaling							
Meditate							
Sauna							
Yoga							
Walk 30 min							
Love Response							
Electronic Detox							
Forgiveness							
Grounding							

Jelena Petkovic PAC MMS

Chapter 32

Next Steps

My dear friends, I hope you have returned to your most beautiful state and rediscovered how beautiful life can be. I hope you have achieved a sense of confidence, knowing you can always fall back on the experience described in this book if you ever get lost again, resetting and nourishing yourself along the way.

We are constantly changing and constantly being challenged and therefore must approach each journey with complete innocence, compassion, and curiosity. Once you understand your dosha, your purpose, your gifts, your passions, and your ideal environment/rhythm/meditations, it will be much easier for you to flourish, to keep your baseline health at a higher level, and to catch yourself sooner if you begin to move away from where you need to be.

My hope for you is that you can use this book as a resource to continually help you find your way back to bliss. You may not need all the meditations and exercises the first time around, but be more open and curious the second or third time around. As you continue to learn about yourself and how you need to be loved, cared for, and nourished, you will create abundance for yourself that will act like a force field of both healing and protection. You too will serve as the healer, teacher or leader in your community.

As easy and beautiful as this all sounds, sometime a self-guided experience is not enough. Sometimes you will need support either because of an existing medical condition or because you need accountability or emotional support. If this is the case, I want to offer a 15-minute consult to anyone who may need advice or wish to work with me. To get your free consult please go to my webpage ABeautifulRx.com/ReturnToBeautiful and sign up for a consult time.

If you want to activate your health and life more sustainably, I have already suggested a more formal meditation practice. As a Chopra Center, certified teacher, I am quite confident in the power of a formal Primordial Sound Meditation practice. My students not only gain the wisdom behind meditation as a form of self-healing but also the confidence to practice long-term and the passion to look forward to expanding their practice with time. The full course is 4 modules long and can be done in a weekend or over a month. I am open for private or group courses over Skype and in person.

As a gift to all my book readers, I am offering a special 25% discount code when purchasing the course. I consider it my dharma (purpose) to teach self-healing techniques that not only help you heal, but prevent disease, and have no side effects. I know that meditation, and especially Primordial Sound Meditation, can serve as a panacea for all types of health issues and help protect you and expand you to the point that you live in effortless bliss despite all obstacles.

For your discount and class scheduling go to ABeautifulRx.com/ReturnToBeautiful and click on "Request Special Primordial Sound Meditation Masterclass." Type in the code RTBactivate16 to receive your discount.

Finally, for all those who are ready for a full immersion of healing and meditation, join me for one of my live workshops or retreats. Check out the current events at ABeautifulRx.com/events/

Proceeds from many of the events will benefit the emotional and mental health of international peace and health organization volunteers supporting refugees and war victims in the Syrian Refugee crisis. I will be taking a small group of healers and mind-body experts to support volunteers who directly impact the health and safety of the thousands of refugees left homeless in Europe.

My dream is to spend at least a quarter of the year helping the healers, teachers and leaders of global health crises, ensuring they are emotionally fit and more resistant to post traumatic stress and compassion fatigue when working with distressed people in need. The healthier the healers and leaders of the world, the more they can transmit peace and love instead of fear and angst.

My wish is for you to join me on my journey to alleviate some of the suffering and spread these vibrations of hope. Please keep a look out for my new non-profit, SoulMedicine Global, and support my events and workshops where I hope to be able to donate all proceeds to this cause so deeply rooted in my heart.

Sat Nam and Blessings to you all!

About the Author

Jelena Petkovic (Indra Shanti Kaur) PAC MMS is a licensed medical practitioner, speaker, and author who specializes in a new medicine known as "integrative Antiaging Medicine," a specialty merging eastern and western medicine tools to prevent disease and premature aging. Jelena blends her expertise in medical detoxification, Ayurveda and digestive health optimization, hormone balancing, and mind-body medicine to help reset and restore people to their most flourishing state of health. In the past 3 years, while working on her doctorate, Jelena has focused her research and practice on mind-body, spiritual and energetic elements as the core focus in patient consultation, diagnosis and treatment. She believes all health issues stem from energetic disequilibrium or misalignment with true self, leading to unhappiness, poor self-care, and disease.

Jelena is passionate about global health and issues surrounding survivors of war and violence, especially the health and future of refugees. Her doctoral work is in Global Health Science and she dedicates research to how to deliver mind-body medicine tools to serve volunteers and field workers of international peace and health organizations working to serve in highly stressful and traumatic situations. 20% of all proceeds of any of Jelena's books, workshops, or events go towards helping the non-profits dedicated to the Syrian refugee cause! Thanks so much for joining her in her pursuit to empower people with free, soulfully beautiful medicine tools.

For some inspiration and support, follow Jelena on Instagram (@heartandsoulmedicine) and share your thoughts and comments on her Facebook page (ABeautifulRx by Jelena Petkovic)

To learn more about Jelena, visit http://www.ABeautifulRx.com

Sat Nam, Blessings and Namaste.

References

Breast Cancer Fund. (2013, February). Breast Cancer and the environment: Prioritizing Prevention: Summary of Recommendations of the interagency breast cancer and environmental research coordinating committee (IBCERRC).

Breast Cancer Fund. (2013, February). Breast Cancer and the environment: Prioritizing Prevention: Summary of Recommendations of the interagency breast cancer and environmental research coordinating committee (IBCERRC).

Breast Cancer Fund. (n.d.a). Chemicals in cosmetics. Retrieved from: http://www.breastcancerfund.org/clear-science/environmental-breast-cancer-links/cosmetics/

Breast Cancer Fund. (n.d.b). Childhood and Adolescence. Retrieved from: http://www.breastcancerfund.org/clear-science/pregnancy-childhood-exposures-breast-cancer-risk/childhood-and-adolescence/

Breast Cancer Fund. (n.d.c). Low Dose Exposures. Retrieved from: http://www.breastcancerfund.org/clear-science/low-dose-exposures-breast-cancer-risk/

Breast Cancer Fund (n.d.d). Prenatal exposure. Retrieved from: http://www.breastcancerfund.org/clear-science/pregnancy-childhood-exposures-breast-cancer-risk/prenatal/

Campaign for Safe Cosmetics. (n.d.a). Chemicals of concern. Retrieved from: http://safecosmetics.org/section.php?id=46

Campaign for Safe Cosmetics. (n.d.b). FAQs for cosmetics companies about The Safe Cosmetics and Personal Care Products Act of 2013. Retrieved from: http://safecosmetics.org/article.php?id=695#about-us

Campaign for Safe Cosmetics (n.d.c). Nanotechnology. Retrieved from: http://safecosmetics.org/article.php?id=307

Campaign for safe Cosmetics. (n.d.d). Pink-ribbon cosmetics. Retrieved from: http://safecosmetics.org/article.php?id=749) p4.

Cohen, S., Janicki-Deverts, D., Turner, R.B., Doyle, W.J. Does hugging provide stress-buffering social support? A study of susceptible to upper respiratory infection and illness. (2015, February) Psychological Science. vol. 26 no. 2 135-147.

Darbre, P.D., Alharrah, A., Miller, W.R., Coldham, N.G., Sauer, M.J., & Pope, G.S. (2004). Concentrations of parabens in human breast tumors. Journal of Applied toxicology, 24(1), 5-13.

Drucker, Peter F. "Smart Goals." The Practice of Management. New York: Harper & Row, 1954.

Environmental Working Group. (n.d) Myths on cosmetic safety. Retrieved from: http://www.ewg.org/skindeep/myths-on-cosmetics-safety/

Friends of the Earth (2009). Brief background information on nanoparticles in sunscreens and cosmetics. Retrieved from: http://safecosmetics.org/downloads/FoE-CSC_NanoCosmetics_factsheet_final_081409.pdf

Kraus, M.W., Huang, C., Keltner, D. Tactile Communication, Cooperation, and Performance: An Ethological Study of the NBA. Emotion, Volume 10, pages 745-749.

Maller, C., Townsend, M., Pryor, A., Brown, P., St. Leger, L. Healthy nature healthy people: 'contact with nature' as an upstream health promotion intervention for populations. Health Promotion International (March 2006) 21(1): 45-54.

Mills, Wilson, Puna, Chinn, Pnatt, Greenberg & Lunde. A simple practice every day: Gratitude and spiritual wellbeing improve mood, energy, self-efficiency and sleep, mediating wellbeing in heart failure patients and clinical outcome.

Social relationships and physiological determinants of longevity across the human life span. Yang, C., Boena, C, Gerkena, B., Ting, L., Kristen Schorppa,B. and Mullan K., Harrisa,b,1.
http://www.pnas.org/content/113/3/578.short

Stahlhut, R.W., van Wijngaarden, E., Dye, T.D., Cook, S., & Swan, S H. (2007). Concentrations of urinary phthalate metabolites are associated with increased waist circumference and insulin resistance in adult US males. Environmental Health Perspectives, 876-882.

Sun, Q., Cornelis, M.C., Townsend, M.K., Tobias, D. K., Eliassen, A.H., Franke, A.A., ... & Hu, F. B. (2014). Association of Urinary Concentrations of Bisphenol A and Phthalate Metabolites with Risk of Type 2 Diabetes: A Prospective Investigation in the Nurses' Health Study (NHS) and NHSII Cohorts. Boston, Massachusetts; Environmental Health Perspectives.

U.S. Food and Drug Administration. (n.d.a.a). Alpha Hydroxy Acids. Retrieved from:
http://www.fda.gov/Cosmetics/ProductsIngredients/Ingredients/ucm107940.htm

U.S. Food and Drug Administration. (n.d.a.b). 'Antibacterial' Soap. In For Consumers. Retrieved from:
http://www.fda.gov/ForConsumers/ConsumerUpdates/ucm378393.htm

U.S. Food and Drug Administration. (n.d.b.c). Eye Cosmetic Safety. Retrieved from: http://www.fda.gov/Cosmetics/ProductsIngredients/Products/ucm137241.htm

U.S. Food and Drug Administration. (n.d.c.d) Is It a Cosmetic, a Drug, or Both? (Or Is It Soap?) http://www.fda.gov/Cosmetics/GuidanceRegulation/LawsRegulations/ucm074201.htm

U.S. Food and Drug Administration. (n.d.d.f). Mercury poisoning linked to skin products. In For Consumers. Retrieved from: http://www.fda.gov/ForConsumers/ConsumerUpdates/ucm294849.htm#2

U.S. Food and Drug Administration. (n.d.f.g). Nail care products. In cosmetic. Retrieved from http://www.fda.gov/Cosmetics/ProductsIngredients/Products/ucm127068.htm#safe

U.S. Food and Drug Administration. (n.d.g.h) Prohibited & restricted ingredients. Retrieved from http://www.fda.gov/cosmetics/guidanceregulation/lawsregulations/ucm127406.htm

U.S. Food and Drug Administration. (n.d.i). Thigh creams. In Products. Retrieved from http://www.fda.gov/cosmetics/

Yang Claire Yang, 578–583, doi: 10.1073/pnas.1511085112 vol. 113 no. 3

SPECIAL GIFT

from Jelena Petkovic

Now that you've read *Return to Beautiful: Journey into Healing, Flourishing Health and Bliss*, you are on your way to creating a life abundant in health, flow and confidence! I'm so excited to share this journey with you, and I know you will continue to not only elevate your life but serve humanity, the planet and all its creatures with a newfound vitality and skill set!!

There's so much confusing information out there about healing both our bodies and spirits. I'm ecstatic to provide you with the most effective integrative methods needed to help you heal, reset and activate your life to the one you were destined to lead!

I have created a special bonus to add to your health toolkit, a new meditation basics video. It will help you establish a regular stress management routine and allow you to access your intuition and creativity with more ease. While this video will be offered for sale to the public, you can claim it for free here:

http://ReturnToBeautiful.com/Gift

The sooner you understand the *Return to Beautiful* strategy, the faster you can begin working on your heart's authentic desires!

I'm in your corner. Let me know if I can help further.

Here's to finding your bliss!

Best,

Jelena Petkovic PAC MMS